THE SPECTER OF AIDS

Before you start to read this book, take this moment to think about making a donation to punctum books, an independent non-profit press,

@ https://punctumbooks.com/support/

If you're reading the e-book, you can click on the image below to go directly to our donations site. Any amount, no matter the size, is appreciated and will help us to keep our ship of fools afloat. Contributions from dedicated readers will also help us to keep our commons open and to cultivate new work that can't find a welcoming port elsewhere. Our adventure is not possible without your support.

Vive la Open Access.

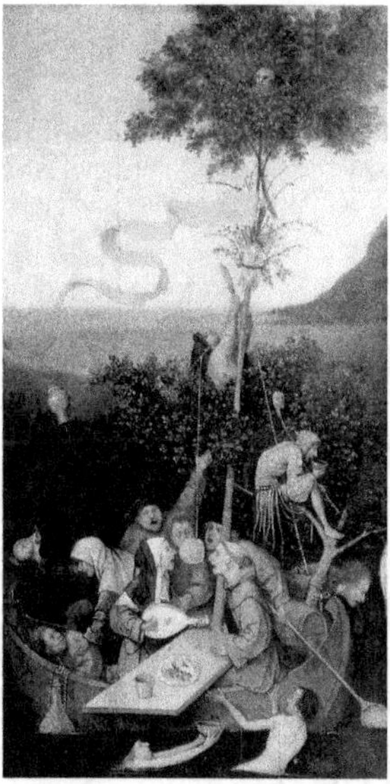

Fig. 1. Detail from Hieronymus Bosch, *Ship of Fools* (1490–1500)

Originally published in Portuguese as *O que é AIDS* (Editora Brasiliense, 1987) and in Spanish as *El fantasma del SIDA* (Puntosur, 1988).
English translation published in 2026 by punctum books, Earth, Milky Way.
https://punctumbooks.com

ISBN-13:978-1-68571-345-4 (paperbound)
ISBN-13: 978-1-68571-346-1 (PDF)
ISBN-13: 978-1-68571-347-8 (EPUB)

DOI: 10.53288/0548.1.00

LCCN: 2026947328
Library of Congress Cataloging Data is available from the Library of Congress

Editing: Vincent W.J. van Gerven Oei and Eileen A. Fradenburg Joy
Book design: Vincent W.J. van Gerven Oei

p. punctumbooks
spontaneous acts of scholarly combustion

HIC SVNT MONSTRA

Néstor Perlongher

The Specter of AIDS

translated by
Jorge Sánchez Cruz

Contents

Contents

Acknowledgments

This project began in 2018 in Chicago, where it was partially supported by the Andrew W. Mellon Foundation and Northwestern University's Program in Critical Theory. I returned to it in 2020 with funds from the American Council of Learned Societies (ACLS) while at the University of Pennsylvania. Along the way, I received comments from Conor Harris. More recently, at UC San Diego, my research assistant Manuel Carrión Lira provided utmost help and insights. In the fall of 2023, after a long search, punctum books gave this text a home. Special commendations to Alejandra Uslenghi who believed, since 2018, on the importance of this translation. Thanks to Roberto Echavarren for permissions to publish this piece in English, to Gabriel Giorgi for writing a beautiful epilogue, and the peer reviewers' supportive commendations. My deepest gratitude to Eileen A. Fradenburg Joy and Vincent W.J. van Gerven Oei at punctum who embraced this translation with deep interest and care.

Translator's Note

Perlongher was a witty and playful poet, writing in a style that also enlivens his scholarship. This translation is an attempt to render such clever and poetic militant writing. All footnotes are mine, including some bibliographic references that complement Perlongher's in-text citations. However, some magazines and journals of the early 1980s that he quotes do not come with bibliographic citations as these sources are not archived, digitized, or have run out of print. Considering the emergency of time, Perlongher was less concerned with citationality and more with demystification of a virus. During the process of translating from the 1988 Spanish edition, the original Portuguese version from 1987 was also consulted.

PROLOGUE

Néstor Perlongher's Afterlives

Jorge Sánchez Cruz

Néstor Perlongher was an unruly figure. He was a militant in Argentina against an authoritarian regime, a sexual dissident, an HIV/AIDS activist, a poet, anthropologist, philosopher, teacher, and a cultural theorist. He wrote about heterosexual masculine desire (prostitution, for instance), sexual subjectivities from the South, homosexuality as a "category," death, transoceanic poetic relations,[1] cruising, medicine and psychiatry, and HIV/AIDS. Perlongher passed away on November 26, 1992, in São Paulo, Brazil. This translation is influenced by his many crafts and skills — his afterlives.

The Specter of AIDS first appeared in 1987 as *O que é AIDS*,[2] a text he wrote and published in Brazil while he lived in exile. A year later, he published the Spanish version, *El fantasma del SIDA*[3] with an additional chapter on AIDS on Argentina that Perlongher disapproved. In trying to keep with the author's desires

1 Néstor Perlongher, *Caribe transplatino: Poesía neobarroca cubana y rioplatense* (Illuminares, 1991).

2 Néstor Perlongher, *O que é AIDS* (Editora Brasilense, 1987).

3 Néstor Perlongher, *El fantasma del SIDA* (Puntosur, 1988). Osvaldo Pedroso translated the Spanish version from the Portuguese, a version Perlongher reworked and which he described as a *trabajo infernal* (infernal labor). See his letter from February 12, 1988 in Néstor Perlongher, *Correspondencia*, ed. Cecilia Palmeiro (Mansalva, 2016), 104–5.

regarding the extra chapter "AIDS in Argentina,"[4] *The Specter of AIDS* appears today as a reincarnated artifact to be read and consulted as new viral contagions emerge to reconfigure the world. The text that you see and read (from within or out loud) is haunting. It diagnoses not only the limits of scientific inquiry and the blind spots of medicine of the 1980s but also exposes how it takes one virus — a pathogen, an infection, a pox, a false categorization (AIDS as GRID) — to make visible the uneven distribution of resources and life possibilities for minority populations. Perlongher's writing left engraved these ghostly concerns not too disconnected from this new millennium.

Néstor's Specter(s)

The text is poetic and at times erotic, especially when Perlongher foregrounds the orifices of the body, the spasms of one's desires, and the bathhouses where sexual intimacies exploded. With an emphasis on the countercultural Brazilian liberatory explosion of letting one's desires run free, a *desbunde*,[5] which diminished, disappeared, or remained secretive with the advent of HIV/AIDS, the text moves across critique and a foregrounding of minoritarian forms of enjoyment. Perlongher was indeed a theorist of desire. In *O negócio de michê* (*The Negotiation of Desire*),[6] he informs us of a subcultural economic exchange between men in Brazilian society. In *Prosa plebeya* (*Plebeian Prose*),[7] which com-

4 In a letter of September 3, 1988, Perlongher states "the press rejected the appendix 'AIDS in Argentina' written by Marcelo Benítez — an interesting perspective — and replaced it without my consent with another piece by Leonardo Moledo that has nothing to do with my point of micropolitical insistence, it is a real sabotage; insulting." Cited in Perlongher, *Correspondencia*, 110.

5 See Cecilia Palmeiro, *Desbunde y felicidad* (Título, 2011).

6 Néstor Perlongher, *O négocio do michê: Prostituição viril em São Paulo* (Editora Brasiliense, 1987).

7 Néstor Perlongher, *Prosa plebeya: Ensayos 1980–1992*, ed. Christian Ferrer and Osvaldo Baigorria (COLIHUE, 1997). See also the English translation: Néstor Perlongher, *Plebeian Prose*, trans. Frances Riddle (Polity Press, 2019).

piles his essays written between 1980 and 1992, the Argentine theorist and anthropologist writes about the embodied forms of yearning of sexual dissidents and their sexual economies as a way to map out and counter the nation-state's panopticon from the social undergrounds, from the favelas to the streets. It is no coincidence that *The Specter of AIDS* begins with the reverberation of how a specter haunts "the streets and the sheets."

Indeed, *The Specter of AIDS* shows how a virus became an aperture for a new administration of embodiment and comportment based on a rhetoric of fear and a discourse of panic that looked to regulate the desires of risk populations. Yet, medicine and normative reason met its limit when attempting to regulate desire. For desire, according to the Argentine theorist, is both a feeling and sensation that moves the minoritarian through the public and private spheres to defy cooption and normativization. *The Specter of AIDS* was written as a desire, a need and an urgency, to change the misconceptions around HIV/AIDS and highlight the un-governmentality of dissident desires.

Perlongher was committed to deconstructing myths and false couplings (HIV with homosexuality or the virus linked to Africa). One could say that he was a Derridean as *The Specter of AIDS* is invested in breaking the missed encounters between science and HIV/AIDS and the false amalgamation between homosexuality and the virus.[8] However, for those who follow Perlongher's work, it is known that he was a fond reader and follower of Gilles Deleuze's philosophy of *lines of flight*.[9] In fact, Perlongher had written "Los devenires minoritarios" (Minoritarian Becomings)[10] as a theoretical formulation of minoritarian

8 In relation to the HIV/AIDS rhetoric and discourse of the time, the dyads of safe/not safe, healthy/unhealthy, and moral/immoral emerged. In this dialectical economy, Perlongher's text appears as an attempt to relieve this dialectic. See Jacques Derrida, *Of Grammatology*, trans. Gayatri Chakravorty Spivak (Johns Hopkins University Press, 1974).

9 Gilles Deleuze and Félix Guattari, *A Thousand Plateaus: Capitalism and Schizophrenia*, trans. Brian Massumi (University of Minnesota Press, 1987).

10 Néstor Perlongher, "Devenires minoritarios," in *El lenguaje libertario*, vol. 2, ed. Christian Ferrer (Nordam, 1991).

life that escapes and shifts away from the restrictive parameters of regimes of power, a kind of disidentification that José Esteban Muñoz would theorize in 1999.[11] For Perlongher, in light of the new biopolitical administration that emerged around HIV/AIDS, minoritarian sexual desires ran fugitive from the constraints of new social codes that made of homosexual and dissident acts and gestures a "moral excess."[12]

As one reads *The Specter of AIDS*, Perlongher deploys analytical inquiries that move away from misinformed narratives and oppressive structures of power. In employing scientific and medical research to further clarify how HIV/AIDS is *not* transmitted, Perlongher's reparative scientific inquiries debunk the falsity of origins of the disease, including, while it may seem general knowledge to today's reader, how an unknown virus was putting to test the validity of science and medicine, the ethical parameters of humanity, and nation states' forms of care. Written in a time of emergency, Perlongher was invested in showing how HIV/AIDS introduced a new methodological arithmetic for the sciences, humanitarian relief, and for the humanities and social sciences overall.

As a social anthropologist and creative writer on sex, gender, and race, in "The Order of Death and the Disorder of Bodies,"[13] Perlongher shows how this viral contagion put forward a new biopolitical and necropolitical administration of human life. The bio and the necro had not become popularized in academic setting, however, Perlongher's analyses show how HIV/AIDS ignited a new barometer for *life* itself, a new order of things that minimized or maximized human value through direct/indirect and implicit/explicit applications of death; how certain bodies, subjects, and populations had better life possibilities as it relates to forms of care available to them while others where inscribed in a landscape of slow death. Although better drugs

11 José Esteban Muñoz, *Disidentifications: Queers of Color and the Performance of Politics* (University of Minnesota Press, 1999).

12 Perlongher, *El fantasma del SIDA*, 79.

13 Ibid., 89–99.

were developed in the the early 1990s, the first antiretroviral therapies (AZT, for instance) were toxic for the human body, not to mention that early cocktails (combination of antiretrovirals) were only accessible to the most well-off, as his contemporary Pedro Lemebel shows in *Loco afán* (*Turbulent Desires*).[14] HIV/AIDS was and is a social "inhibitor" for the survival of the classed and racialized populations in the Global South.

Moreover, the social was tied to the moral, and according to Perlongher, HIV/AIDS made morality anew. Doctor recommendations created a new form a normalization, a corrective and regulatory practice, veiled with moralizing predicaments, a moral compass tied to the regulation and normalization of subjects linked to the errors of medical science and social misinformation. *The Specter of AIDS* makes the reader wonder when and how these administrative vectors are veiled when a patient seeks medical care. And when is such moralizing gaze re-actualized when seeking HIV/AIDS and reproductive care? Could the text be read as one more antecedent of how viral panic, illness, and pathogenic contamination shape the social, medical, racial, and ethical configurations of our twenty-first century?

Viral Intimacies

The HIV/AIDS pandemic is not over. The residues of the 1980s, its misconceptions and falsities, along with who has access to retroviral care are still dire issues across the globe. *The Specter of AIDS* tells us that the virus created new intimate relations amidst these circumstances. On the one hand, these intimacies can become violent (antithetical) between seropositivity with social agents, between medicine and science with minority groups, and through discourses that negatively affect specific groups suspected of being carriers. However, affirmative intimate connections can also emerge through the ethical responsibility for those in need, creating community forms of care and political activism and militancy for the nurturing of the many

14 Pedro Lemebel, *Loco afán: Crónicas de sidario* (Editorial Anagrama, 1986).

lives being lost to HIV/AIDS. In some cases, "risky" sexual practices created subcultural forms of kin through an embrace of the virus as a connecting vector, such as in breeding cultures or bug chasing practices. The virus created and yet diminished different forms of intimacies with others as seen in the movements across the Americas and beyond.

In the twenty-first century, viral emergencies unveil new forms of intimate relations, or rather reproduce the intimacies seen with HIV/AIDS. The catastrophic virus of COVID-19 that appeared in 2019, also known as the Coronavirus, caused by the SARS-CoV-2 virus, created what Perlongher mentions as the "re-ordering of bodies." COVID-19 created panic, social paranoia, and xenophobia in the United States and elsewhere. Its "origins" were taken to China by an uninformed press and racist journalism. These origins became contested and deconstructed, just as Perlongher throws off the "origins" of HIV/AIDS that demonized — and "shamed" — gay culture and which also "blamed" African populations.[15] With COVID-19, Chinese and Asian populations in general became falsely coupled with the disease as its purported carriers, creating a racialized biopolitical distribution of peoples that also racially codified the borders worldwide: who can enter countries such as the United States, and who are excluded for being potential threats to public health (a discourse normalized in the US under a guise of "public safety" and "national security").[16] Antithetical intimacies arose through racial discrimination in the United States, violence against minority groups, and even calls for the expulsion of certain bodies. More insidiously were the intimate intricacies of hegemonic entities — the pharmaceutical industries and empire-colonial states — that prevented, even halted, the access to the first developed vaccines against COVID-19. This in turn created a process of forced deaths and even slow mechanisms of letting die across the hemisphere, like the many lives lost

15 Perlongher, *El fantasma del SIDA*, 41–52.

16 "DHS Responds: Coronavirus (COVID-19)," *Department of Homeland Security*, https://www.dhs.gov/archive/coronavirus.

to HIV/AIDS in the 1980s and 1990s due to the inefficiencies of governments to act rapidly. This, however, did not prevent the emergence of positive intimate relations, as many people assembled food distribution, the enforcement of masks and social distancing, monetary chains of support, and affirmative affective engagements when COVID-19 threatened or took someone's life.[17]

Perlongher's observations of how a virus creates a "regime of bodies" speaks of recent viral arrivals.[18] Viruses come to reproduce, or reinforce, certain ideals of embodiment tied to racialized and gendered paradigms. Take for instance, the specter of pox as the monkeypox virus. The recent surge within the last two–three years has renewed the false ideas that homosexuality and Blackness are the sources of infectious viral diseases. Monkeypox, like HIV/AIDS and COVID-19 (and their many variants), has also much to do with encounters. The encounters with the limits of and the dispersion of (misinformed) knowledge, as well as with differential embodiment, as most of the times monkeypox reveals severe corporeal signs, led to the call to diminish antithetical proximities with those narrativized as the "originators" and "spreaders" of the virus. Monkeypox, like COVID-19, is therefore also a litmus test for the world, posing the questions of how forms of aid will respond to embrace the affected other(s) and if health programs, political discourse, dominant rhetoric, and public policy will come to emphasize a renewed learned approach to viral threats that make certain bodies and peoples more vulnerable than others. The limited availability of the monkeypox vaccine (mpox) and its treatment (Tpoxx) made the uneven distribution of resources, the access to health facilities, and the lack of properly trained medical personnel that can provide alleviating and ethical encounters once more apparent.

---

17 Elsewhere I have written on how intimate relational encounters assemble communities of aliveness and ethical embrace of differential otherness. See Jorge Sánchez Cruz, "Intimacy, Relationality, Repair: AIDS, Mexico, and the Case of Agustín Martínez Castro," *Journal of Latin American Cultural Studies* 34, no. 1 (2025): 47–73.

18 Perlongher, *El fantasma del SIDA*, 89.

Intimacies — negative and positive — arise in the context of viral threats.

Forty years after its original inception, *The Specter of AIDS* reappears to shed light on how HIV/AIDS exposes the horrors and inequalities of a time. It also foregrounds how unregulated desires of minority subcultures conjoined to enjoyment and community organizing can still flourish in times of catastrophe. HIV/AIDS nonetheless is a haunting ghost as it materialized into structures, myths, and stigmas hard to completely undo today. Its specter alerts us that sometimes it takes just a single virus to make apparent how fucked up the world is and can be for the more disenfranchised of the Earth.

San Diego, California
October 25, 2024

The Specter of AIDS

Introduction

A specter is haunting the streets, the sheets, and the flirts: the specter of AIDS. Merely mentioning the foreboding acronym (the acronym for Acquired Immunological Deficiency Syndrome) is enough to provoke a morbid mixture of fear and curiosity.

In the beginning, paranoia seemed restricted to North American homosexuals. On the West coast of the United States, in the city of San Francisco, to be precise — the epicenter of the potent "sexual revolution" that shook the mucus of the West and threatened to subvert the castes that ruled during two thousand years of Christianity— between 1980 and 1981, there were a series of strange deaths.

It was referred to as the "gay cancer," the "pink plague." In fact, the first extraofficial designation given — GRID (Gay Related Immune Deficiency) — bore the same sort of originary link between illness and homosexuality (until recently, of course, homosexuality was itself considered an illness). However, the emergence of cases in other population sites shifted the orientation of medical research and gave the illness a definite name.

What is AIDS? Although scientific knowledge has made extensive progress, this evil is still cloaked in mystery. We know it is transmitted through sexual contact or blood transfusion. This is not — like some moralists pretend to claim — a "homosexual sickness": eventually, the virus that causes it can be transmitted

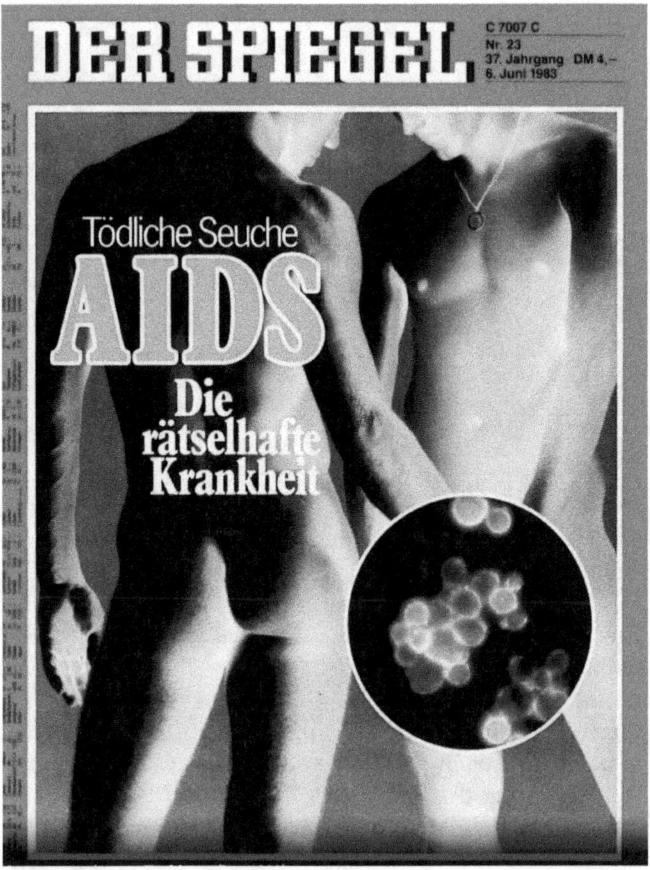

Figure 1.1. AIDS in 1983: Homosexual paranoia makes the most important headlines in the world.

by and to any person. Once triggered, the sickness is practically fatal. To date, there is no known cure for AIDS.

The commotion provoked by AIDS appears somewhat disproportionate in relationship to its real statistical impact. In spite of some apocalyptic projections, which even predict humanity's extinction, currently, AIDS is less fatal than other, well-known illnesses — malnutrition, circulatory problems, cancer, intra-hospital infections, etcetera. There is a much better chance of dying struck by a car in the street than as a consequence of AIDS. But the horror of bodies that become contaminated and die is all the more terrifying when one intuits that, at the heart of this agony's contortions, lay spasms of pleasure.

Just as AIDS, from its beginning, transcended the particularity of the victims' pains to extend throughout the "ghettos" corridors as a powerful mechanism of moralization and control, born of waves of panic, this specter seems to have abandoned the bounds of the minoritarian circuits where it lurked to also terrify heterosexual life. Initially seen as a "homosexual disease," AIDS has been announced as a threat to the nuclear family.

The iconography of this shift is easily traced by flipping through the pages of the weekly news (fig. 1.1). The German magazine *Der Spiegel* (*The Mirror*) printed, on the cover of its June, 1983 edition, an image of two naked men, one with his genitalia circled and magnified to show microscopic germs (death symbolized by the precise object of desire);[1] three years later, in December of 1986, the same publication substituted these two athletic youth for a heterosexual couple, set against a skeletal Cupid, aiming his poisonous arrows (fig. 1.1).

The panic caused by the virus is not as unheard of as has been said; similar nightmares were provoked throughout history by successive plagues. Nor is discrimination a novelty. During the medieval plagues, Jews were persecuted and accused of deliberately contaminating the water, or because their mere existence

1 The 1987 Brazilian version includes an image of the magazine cover of *Der Spiegel* that reads "Deadly Plague. AIDS. The Mysterious Illness." Perlongher adds his own subheading under the image.

was considered an attack on Divine Will, who, offended, sought revenge. Similarly, in 1985, a story appears concerning the expulsion of a hairdresser from the city of Araguari, in Minas Gerais, accused of plunging maliciously into a club's pool, without even being sick of HIV/AIDS.[2] It seems that heavenly arguments have not changed much.

An illness related to sexuality touches on a particularly sensitive point for contemporary society, so concerned with hygiene and bodily care. In the case of AIDS, to such a loaded stigma, a sign of so many of the social order's rules, a further complication is added, derived from the possibility of blood-borne transmission. At this point, a new question emerges: Despite the everyday practice of transfusions, would the fear of mixing blood not retain, in the social imaginary, the force of its atavistic symbolism? The age of Nazism wielding the principles of blood purity to establish an Aryan race is not too far gone. We might sketch out a somber similarity between the current decline of the *sexual revolution*—crowning a voracious epoch of contestatory experiences—and the wild madness of the 1920s and 1930s, the *Daring Years,* preceding the twin horrors of fascism and of war.

The emergence of AIDS puts into play a variety of articulations that need not only be limited to the field of medical sciences. More than ever, it has become necessary to attend to the social and sexual repercussions of this unsettling problem, which concerns bodily relationships and their affects.

It is worth noting that, due to the simple fact of AIDS being a new disease, an increasing body of, sometimes contradictory, information enters into circulation on a daily basis. Under these conditions, few absolute truths can be discerned; statements—including the medical—cannot hide, at the moment, their provisional nature. Insofar as this book is affected by these circumstances, the interpretations and hypotheses here

2 Perlongher notes this example of a hairdresser falling into a pool and being banished from a town in Brazil to show the tenuous developing and false coupling between homosexuality to HIV/AIDS.

dispensed are conditioned by this provisional state. Far from avoiding polemics, the idea is, on the contrary, to complicate them; only the broadest possible discussion will radiate the more lucid perspectives we need to understand and confront this complex issue.

The Illness

AIDS — Acquired Immunodeficiency Syndrome. This name bundles a series of medical concepts often difficult to understand. To better comprehend it, what follows is a clarification of each separate term that the acronym encompasses.

Syndrome: a set of symptoms that occur more or less simultaneously, with one or various common causes. AIDS is defined as a syndrome because it lacks a single manifestation; on the contrary, it is characterized by the appearance of various, simultaneous, and ongoing infections that "conceal" the true illness.

Immunodeficiency: this is a deficiency of the immune system.[1] Immunity is the organism's capacity to recognize and destroy "attacking invaders." But why deficiency? Because the peculiarity of this illness is that it causes this system to cease functioning, exposing the organism to a multiplicity of infectious agents. While most are normally harmless, they can attain, in said conditions, a harmful state of development. AIDS is precisely an illness of the immune system, that triggers an overall collapse of the organism's defenses.

Acquired: there are hereditary forms of immunological deficiency. In the case of AIDS, immunodeficiency is acquired

1 While Perlongher utilizes the term *immunological system*, the term used here, *immune system*, reflects contemporary terminology.

through contamination; that is, an infectious agent penetrates the organism through blood, sperm, or through certain discharges found in another hosting orgamism.

Contending Terminologies

Once understood and described by medicine as a disturbance of the immunological system, the next step was discovering the cause of this new illness. In the United States, there was initially a discussion about whether the causative agent was singular (the so-called *unifactorial theory*) or a confluence of sanitary and social factors (*multifaceted theory*)— a significant polemic in the history of medicine. The unifactorial theory would gain visibility when it was discovered that AIDS, as will be revealed further on, is caused by a virus. It is worth noting, however, one of the multifactorial theses: that the illness was not a consequence of a new infectious agent, but rather that patients' symptoms arise from exposure to extremely harmful "biological environments," characterized by different sets of venereal diseases and simultaneous infections.

Scientists had thought that some forms of cancer could have been caused by a virus. Viruses are miniscule agents (a tenth of a thousandth of a millimeter) unable to survive independently, for which they require a parasitic relationship with another's living cells.

The American doctor Robert Gallo was able to isolate the virus causing a very rare form of leukemia (one which, at the same time, had already been spreading in the US South). Gallo named this virus HTLV-1 (Human T Cell Leukemia Virus, that is, a human leukemic virus that attacks T cells; these are in charge of, among other functions, immunological defense), and believed himself to be, in the case of AIDS, close to a variant of this evil.

But it would be the other side of the Atlantic where the virus was discovered. Credit for the discovery must be given to the team at the Institute Pasteur in Paris, directed by Doctor Montagnier. By performing a lymph node biopsy on a homosexual patient, who would not end up developing the illness, in 1983, a *completely new virus* was baptized as LAV (Lymphadenopathy Associated Virus, that is, a virus associated with the diseases of the lymphatic system, where the lymph glands are found).[2]

Meanwhile, American scientists continued their research and, in 1984, were able to artificially isolate the virus in a laboratory. Gallo's discovery is promoted as "a miracle of medicine and of American science." [3]

Gallo's team gave the virus their own name, HTLV-III (Human T Lymphotropic Virus Type III).[4] Recently there was an attempt to resolve the disagreement in terminologies by proposing a new designation for the virus: HIV (Human Immunodeficiency Virus).[5]

The Immune System

To explain what the AIDS virus is and how it acts, one must discuss the human immune system a bit further.

This system has at least two major functions. The first relates to the *external* environment, its inhabitants, and their aggres-

2 Perlongher utilizes glands instead of nodes. Both are the same and both play a vital role in fighting off infections. See Luc Montagnier, "A History of HIV Discovery," *Science* 298, no. 5599 (2002): 1727–28.

3 Perlonger is referring to an anonymous opinion piece from *The New York Times* where Secretary Margaret Heckler mentions "Today we add another miracle to the long honor roll of American medicine and science." See "A Viral Competition over AIDS," *The New York Times*, April 26, 1984, 22.

4 See Robert C. Gallo et al., "Frequent Detection and Isolation of Cytopathic Retro-viruses (HTLV-III) from Patients with AIDS and at Risk for AIDS," *Science* 224, no. 4648 (1984): 500–503. Their term is associated with their two previous, related findings.

5 It is now agreed that Montaigne's team first isolated IV and Gallo's group is given credit for discovering that the virus causes AIDS, since, in the publication of the former's discovery they mentioned that whether HIV causes AIDS "remains to be determined." Gallo is also credited for much of the science, including developing a lab technique for the growing of T cells. In 1986, the French and US presidents agreed on dropping both terms in favor of HIV.

sions. The second is relegated to the *interiority of the individual,* its own organism, protecting it from diverse morbid processes that develop silently. Together they form extensive, dual lines of defense.

The external is constituted by the skin and the mucus membranes that cover, for instance, the respiratory tracts, including all secretions. If this barrier happens to be traversed by invasive bodies, which then enter the blood stream, then the second defense system, the interior, will activate a set of specialized immune cells.

Although it may seem that these two, major functions are separate, they depend, above all, on a central component of the specialized immune system, a type of white blood cell called the "helper" T4 lymphocyte.[6] The function of the "helper" T lymphocyte could be compared to that of a central computer, feeding all other terminals while emitting information to the remaining components of the immune system, the latter allowing organization of the organism's defenses against attacks by foreign bodies. This entire process takes place in the bloodstream.

These components or terminals are significantly varied. Some, like the B lymphocytes, produce antibodies, protein molecules present in the bloodstream that help eliminate unfamiliar agents from the organism, detecting and "labeling" them. Hence, as regards the AIDS virus, there are specific types of antibodies produced that signal and keep a record of its presence.

How, then, does the relationship between B lymphocytes and T4 lymphocyte "helpers" usually function? When the organism is in contact with the measles virus, for example, the B lymphocytes, after receiving orders from the T lymphocyte "helpers," start to produce antibodies against that microorganism. Once the risk has passed and there is no need to maintain the production of antibodies, it is also the T lymphocyte "helpers" that

6 Otherwise known as the Helper T cell or the CD4+ cell, a key mediator of the immune function.

send information to another type of T8 lymphocytes ("suppressors"), ordering them to cease the attack.

The Virus

The AIDS virus attacks in a particularly malignant way because it works against the very cells in charge of immunological defenses. Once the virus penetrates the bloodstream, it seeks hosting cells (as it cannot develop on its own, it relies on the parasitism of specific types of cells). The AIDS virus has, in fact, a special affinity with "helper" T4 lymphocytes.

Once the virus is able to penetrate into the cell, it may well remain indefinitely dormant. However, for unknown reasons, by taking advantage of the activation of the "helper" T4 lymphocyte's cellular machinery, it is capable of massive self-reproduction and multiplication. While the cell merely splits in two, the virus is reproduced millions of times, transforming the cell into a veritable power plant for its own destruction. Once multiplied, the virus enters other cells, preferably T lymphocytes and, secondarily, some brain cells. Herein dissemination begins.

The infected cells can be stimulated — for example, by a "common" infection — to increase the multiplication of the virus. As such, new infections in the organisms already besieged by LATV/HTLV-III can contribute to the worsening of AIDS.

Since there are millions of T4 lymphocytes, some time elapses before the immune system is compromised. But once this process is triggered, the latter will progressively be taken out of combat. At a given moment, no cells will remain to combat any infections which the patient may contract.

The Symptoms

The ubiquity of the symptoms — they can take so many forms! — makes them uncertain: swelling of the lymph nodes, fatigue without cause, involuntary weight loss, intermittent fever, diarrhea, and persistent coughs.

These clinical signs are not unique to AIDS, as some can correspond to other illnesses, like tuberculosis. It is uncommon to suspect AIDS if dealing with a light fever, sweating, and diarrhea, all too common for a gamut of diseases.

Suspicion becomes appropriate given the duration and extreme complexity of symptoms that resist other explanations.

Moreover, most manifestations of the AIDS virus are benign. More than half of those who come into contact with the virus develop neither symptoms nor illness. Some could be called healthy (or asymptomatic) carriers of the illness who, without manifesting it, bear the virus and may eventually transmit it. For the time being, there is no determinate way how and at which moment such transmission becomes possible.

The Development of Symptoms

Two to six weeks after the virus enters the organism, one can observe, in twenty percent of cases, some clinical manifestations. Among them, mononucleosis syndrome: fevers, the inflammation of lymph nodes, and some redness on the skin. These symptoms disappear spontaneously after about ten days; their presence indicates nothing in relation to AIDS's eventual severity.

During the following three months, after penetration by the virus, the organism will produce the antibodies that signal contact with a foreign body.

Of the infected persons, only a minority will develop the most serious forms of this evil. Some will go on to present lesser manifestations, often not particularly apparent, and others present certain secondary symptoms, a sort of "benign tableau" that does not generally evolve to fatal forms. These tableaus may be grouped according to two principal configurations: Chronic Lymphadenopathy Syndrome and, more importantly, ARC or AAS (AIDS Related Complex, for the Americans; AIDS Associated Syndrome, for the French).

Chronic Lymphadenopathy Syndrome or PGL (Persistent Generalized Lymphadenopathy) refers to discomfort of the lymphatic organs. PGL is characterized by augmentation in the volume of the lymphatic ganglia, which can reach abnormal dimensions, frequently greater than a centimeter in diameter, in different parts of the body, most often in the neck or the armpits. This augmentation can persist for months or years: neither their size nor duration indicate a hypothetical evolution toward lethal forms of AIDS. The inflammation of the lymph nodes is common in a wide range of infections: only upon observing a clear augmentation in volume, unattributable to other causes, can one establish a relationship to the presence of the AIDS virus.

AIDS Associated Syndrome or ARC

Within this tableau, we observe minor afflictions, most often fungal infections, also known as *muguet,* which appear on the face, nails, or mouth. ARC can also manifest as a prolonged fever, above thirty-eight degrees, for a period of several weeks; as unintentional weight-loss that exceeds ten percent of body mass; and as an abundance of night sweats that oblige a change of bedsheets.

Even purplish lesions may appear — small hemorrhagic spots on the legs — which correlate to an excessive defense response by the organism, increasing disorderly production of antibodies, which turn against blood platelets. But nor does this signal AIDS: these symptoms do not necessarily evolve toward a complete collapse of organic defenses.

The two frameworks described are provoked by the AIDS virus. However, they are not, strictly speaking, AIDS. What is happening is that the majority of virus's manifestations are, as stated, benign. Only when malignant manifestations appear can one discuss AIDS stricto sensu.

AIDS *stricto sensu*

What happens to those who develop the illness? Given the sharp fall in the organism's defenses, generally inoffensive germs take advantage of the moment to invade the organism. Opportunistic infections then appear, so called because they can only develop in these favorable conditions.

At a first glance, when the virus's spread is not yet severe, opportunistic infections are limited to the mucous membranes (genital herpes, oral thrush) or become visible through ongoing, minor, yet persistent infections, such as sinusitis, furuncles, etcetera.

As AIDS advances, opportunistic diseases multiply. They might affect the lungs, the digestive tract, the nervous system, and can even access the skin. At the neurological level, prolonged headaches may constitute an indicative symptom. One may also detect a treatable, if caught early, case of toxoplasmosis.

One of the most common illnesses is a serious form of pneumonia, caused by the parasite *Pneumocystis carinii.* Moreover, some forms of cancer begin to appear, such as Kaposi Sarcoma.

Kaposi Sarcoma

One of AIDS's most well-known manifestations is Kaposi Sarcoma, an illness with its own history. It seems a banal illness: small, purplish plaques, which traditionally appear on the lower body. Initially discovered in the Jewish "ghettos" of central Europe, it was attributed to promiscuity. There, the Viennese doctor, Moritz Kaposi (in reality, a pseudonym) discovered the illness and gave it his name. This illness, according to Professor Jean-Paul Escande's description from the Pasteur Institute of Paris, "is at the limits of cancer."[7] Rarely lethal, it was still considered an oddity.

In this century, a somewhat more aggressive, African variant of Kaposi Sarcoma was discovered, characterized by the emer-

7 While there is no direct source for Perlongher's citation, he followed Escande's research on the connection between HIV/AIDS with cancer from his early discoveries in Isabelle Gorin et al., "Kaposi's Sarcoma without the U.S. or 'Popper' Connection," *The Lancet* 319, no. 8277 (1982): 908, to a more clear connection in N. Dupin et al., "Herpesvirus-like DNA with Mediterranean Kaposi's Sarcoma," *The Lancet* 345 no. 8952 (1995): 761–62.

gence of real tumors, ulcerated lesions, and voluminous lymph nodes.

The minoritarian legacy of this illness was easily transmitted to homosexuals. Thus, AIDS was initially considered "Kaposi for gays" and, unfortunately, nicknamed the "gay cancer," even by California's homosexual dailies themselves.

However, the Kaposi associated with AIDS assumes a more violent form: a generalized outbreak that drags on for months, attacking the internal organs and the face. Average survival is barely two years.

The collapse of the immune system caused by AIDS can also favor the proliferation of other types of cancer, such as lymphomas (tumors developed throughout the lymph nodes) that mainly affect the brain.

AIDS is, without a doubt, not a cancer. But it does open the door to a diverse set of malignant tumors.

Transmission

The AIDS virus is transmitted through sperm, vaginal secretions, or through blood. These substances can be habitually transferred between people; in sperm and blood, the virus lives inside the cells, with some limits on its survivability.

AIDS is a minimally contagious illness, relatively speaking; its causative agent dies when it comes into contact with air or alcohol. The most common way of acquiring it is through sexual contact. But it can also be transmitted through a transfusion of blood containing infected cells, carrying them from one individual to another. This explains cases of contamination through blood transfusions or through needle sharing by drug addicts.

Signs of the virus have also been found in saliva and in tears. However, the possibilities of the virus being transported through these organic liquids are scarce (in the worst of cases, it would be necessary for the saliva or the tears to enter the bloodstream through an open wound). A polemic between the Americans and the French as regards kissing has thus been revived. While, for the scientists of the Pasteur Institute, contamination through these means is less probable, their more cautious North American rivals tend to discourage prolonged kissing.

Unverified sources also suggest that AIDS could be transmitted by a mosquito. But it would be quite difficult, critics of this farfetched theory have adduced, to conceive of a mosquito being capable of identifying their victims' sexual preferences.

There is, in some ways, a hierarchy of risk. Anal sex is particularly dangerous, as the penis's friction against the rectal walls can produce microscopic wounds, through which the virus could enter the bloodstream. Following this reasoning, it is presumed that the passive individual would be more at risk during anal penetration than the active one.[8] The latter, however, could also be at risk, since the virus may also penetrate through the penis's microlesions.

The mucus membrane that covers the vaginal cavity is also less fragile than the rectum. However, diffusion of AIDS in Africa, predominantly among heterosexuals, reawakens doubts.

Precise data does not exist which would allow for evaluating the true risks of transmitting the AIDS virus after oral–genital contact (like fellatio). Accordingly, possibilities of contamination would be linked to the roughness of the interaction. The sources consulted do not register the presence of LAV/HTLV-III in urine or in fecal matter. Any oral–anal contact tends to be discouraged, even if the possibility of contagion — discounting any wounds to these organs — is still not clearly established.

There exists uncertainty around the probability that the virus could be transmitted through tattoos, orthodontic treatments, or acupuncture done with inadequately sterilized instruments. Out of caution, it is recommended that intimate objects, like toothbrushes, shaving blades, nail clippers, etc. used by AIDS patients not be used by other persons.

---

8 In more vernacular terms, those in a passive role (bottom) would be more susceptible to viral or STI transmissions than those in an active role (top).

What Transmits AIDS

Proven contagion
— Anal sex
— Vaginal sex
— Contact with sperm
— Blood transfusions
— Unsterilized Syringes
— Intrauterine Infection (when the fetus contracts the illness through the mother)

Possible contagion
— Oral–anal contact
— Oral–genital contact
— Prolonged kissing
— Acupuncture or tattooing with unsterilized instruments
— Shaving blades or toothbrushes used by the ill
— Unsterilized nail clippers, scissors, or blades
— Unsterilized orthodontic or surgical instruments
— Licking of wounds
— Contacting menstrual blood
— Tears (minimally probable)

Not Transmitting AIDS
— Air
— Water from pools
— Sauna vapors
— Showers
— Bus seats
— Doorknobs
— Toilets
— Handshakes
— Kisses on the face (avoiding wounds)
— Food
— Cutlery
— Plates
— Bedsheets

— Paper money
— Donating blood (with sterilized instruments)

How AIDS Is Not Transmitted

An infinite set of myths manage to explain the most fantastical forms of AIDS awareness. Ranging from the refusal of "social" kissing, a handshake, to even not touching doorknobs nor using toilets where the ill have allegedly been. Equally mythical is the belief in the possibility of contamination in public pools or the bedding of motels. The danger of transmission through cups, cutlery, plates, etc., even if only washed superficially, is null. Paper currency is also not dangerous.

Although the dissemination of the illness has created a sharp drop in blood donors, donating does not offer any danger of contamination, as long as the instruments used are correctly sterilized.

The Test

Diagnosing the presence of the AIDS virus in the blood is a difficult and expensive task. The most common serological (blood work) tests allow for the direct inference of the virus's passage through the blood by detecting antibodies; that is, molecules capable of "marking" the virus.

This test sets out from the principle that infections by the AIDS virus are products of unknown agents entering into the organism. As a response, specific antibodies are produced to fight them. These antibodies remain active for a prolonged period and function to signal the virus's presence.

The most commonly used test is called ELISA.[9] The presence of the antibody, which reveals the virus's existence, is revealed

9 ELISA is also called EIA, an enzyme-linked immunosorbent assay commonly used to detect antibodies, antigens, and proteins. It is administered not only for HIV-testing, but also in pregnancy tests and for measurements of cytokines.

by a colored reaction. In this case, it is a seropositive reaction, which is then confirmed by a new test.

Nonetheless, a seropositive result does not necessarily indicate that the person tested has AIDS, only that its organism had some type of contact with the virus and consequently produced those specific antibodies. If an individual with a seropositive result does not show any other symptoms, it is not possible to know whether he is a "healthy" carrier of the virus.

When the seropositive result is combined with symptoms characteristic of infection by the AIDS virus, other, more complex tests are performed—immunofluorescence,[10] radioimmunoassay,[11] radioimmunoprecipitation,[12] and the Western Blott[13]—in order to detect, with certainty, the presence of the virus.

The ELISA test is not entirely effective, as it may produce false positives or false negatives. If a person has a positive result, it does not mean they have AIDS, but—we insist—only that they possess the respective antibodies. It is calculated that no more than fifteen percent of the seropositive results ultimately contract the illness.

In spite of the ongoing medical pronouncements in favor of a type of generalized, anti-HTLV-III testing, other voices from within the medical field advise against the risks of its random application. In an article titled "HTLV-III: Should Testing Everyone Be Routine?" the authors note that the arguments in favor

---

10 Immunofluorescence is a technique used for light microscopy with a fluorescent microscope, used primarily for microbiological samples, that is, a procedure to detect antigens.

11 Radioimmunoassay is an immunoassay that used radiolabeled molecules in a step-by-step structuration of immune complexes. It is a very sensitive in vitro technique that measures concentrations of substances. It also measures antigen levels by use of antibodies.

12 Radioimmunoprecipitation or the RIPA (Radio-Immunoprecipitation Assay) buffer is "essential for the rapid, efficient cell lysis and solubilization of proteins from both adherent and suspension-cultured mammalian cells."

13 The Western Blott is used in molecular biology and immunogenetics to detect specific proteins in a sample of tissues.

of systematic application of tests to detect antibodies proper to the AIDS virus are not as logical as they seem.[14] Insofar as there is still no known effective vaccine or treatment, random testing would bring, as a product of a "seropositive" result, considerable risks for patients as individuals: psychological damage, both emotional and existential, as already suffered by numerous patients who, believing they had AIDS, entered a profound crisis. The possibility of reversing this psychological state is quite low, given the panic that tends to invade patients. These effects do not provoke the slightest concern among those promoting generalized testing, who are predisposed to painting apocalyptic scenes. Sensitized for similar reasons as the immunocompromised, members of the Carioca homosexual group Pink Triangle refused the free testing offered by a clinical team, distrusting the presumed benefits the tests might offer.

Beyond its doubtful utility, generalized testing of an entire population — and consequently, the internment of the seropositive, ill or not, until the discovery of a cure (a proposal made in San Pablo by a North American doctor proclaiming the end of the world as a result of the spread of AIDS) would be a fabulous commercial enterprise. It is not all delusional to see how behind many alarmist apostles lay excessive interests in exploiting the vast spectrum of AIDS-related enterprises.

Hope for the Cure

There is currently no known cure for AIDS. The mortality rate for people who reach the final stage of the illness oscillates between eighty-five and a hundred percent. Medicine is limited to treating, with mixed fortunes, the opportunistic infections or emerging cancers — an attempt to delay, as much as possible, what is a supposedly inexorable death. A common risk shared by most of these "severe" illnesses: a more complicated death and greater agony.

14 David Miller et al., "HTLV-III: Should Testing be Routine?," *British Medical Journal* 45, no. 6525 (1986): 941–43.

Some opportunistic diseases, like pneumonia (provoked by *Pneumocystis carinii*), meningitis (caused by *Cryptococcus neoformans*), and encephalitis (provoked by *Toxoplasma gondii*), disappear slowly but regain ground shortly after a halt in medication. For other infections there is practically no treatment, as is the case with cytomegalovirus,[15] the Epstein-Barr virus,[16] and polyoma (which provokes a progressive, multifocal leukoencephalopathy).

Kaposi Sarcoma is also difficult to treat, but in forty percent of extant cases showing initial stages of the illness and in patients with no concurrent opportunistic diseases we see some involution through the application of interferon or chemotherapy (although the latter facilitates a surge in opportunistic infections).

There has been some experimentation with drugs that specifically target the retrovirus — HPA 23, suramin, ribavirin, Alpha interferon, and AZT (azidothymidine) — yet the reduction of viral production as a result of their application is generally temporary and inefficacious for those in later stages, with the risk of also causing complex collateral effects. In reality, medicine has not progressed far on the slippery battlefield against the virus.

There is much speculation as regards the possibility of a vaccine against AIDS. Occasionally, medical representatives and the mass media machine chime in, giving risky, vague timelines: one, three, fifteen years. It is true that scientists' endeavors are intense. However, detailing the reiterated attempts would require an excessively technical digression. It is fitting to simply sketch out the difficulties that indefinitely postpone such a hope's realization.

In the first place, we are talking about an extremely mutative virus (the protein layer that covers it is what is transmuted). One possible route is bypassing the creation of specific antibodies. However, the virus can coexist, as seen in the tests, with anti-

15 The cytomegalovirus is also known as herpes. Once the virus enters the body, it may be suppressed but lays dormant.

16 The Epstein-Barr virus is another variant of herpes.

bodies designed to neutralize it. Additionally, it has been difficult to find an animal model to run experimental tests. The closest would be the chimpanzee, which could perhaps be contaminated by the virus, but the infection is almost imperceptible in the organism. Aside from that, sustaining them is also quite costly.

Risks and Recommendations

In the absence of a cure, medical recommendations are limited to the plane of prevention and avoiding practices considered dangerous. We list a few medical and paramedical suggestions:

— reducing the number of partners:[17] by the law of probability, the most promiscuous would be the more exposed to contagion;
— to avoid contact with sperm;
— the use of prophylactics: a resource demonstrated to be effective against other viruses—latex impedes their crossing. If not well placed, it could rip, or semen can overflow. It is recommended to also use lubricant and it must be placed on the penis when erect. Some spermicides were shown to be effective in in vitro experiments, but doubts still persist;
— using individual, disposable syringes, recommended for users of intravenous drugs;
— abstaining from acts considered at higher risk of contamination (according to the "Transmission" section): anal and vaginal sex, oral–genital and oral–anal encounters, and all that imply mixing of secretions.

Far from being "innocent," these recommendations spring from a certain medical model of bodily practices that has a troubled relationship with specific uses of the body. But before discuss-

17 Perlongher uses here the French word *partenaires* (partners).

ing these ideological foundations, it is necessary to present the controversy (not less ideological) regarding the origins of AIDS.[18]

18 This last sentence is not part of the Spanish version, but it is found in the Portuguese. It is included here as it provides a transition to the next chapter, emphasizing how controversies concerning origins can also be ideological.

The Fable of Origins

The origin of AIDS is foggy. Clinical uncertainty drives the proliferation of myths, the limits of wisdom of which are, in contemporary society, somewhat diffuse.

The first alleged cases of AIDS were documented in the south of Japan in September 1979 and, five months later, in the Caribbean. In light of recent data, it is somewhat doubtful whether they were really cases of AIDS. They could perhaps have been cases of a rare form of leukemia, whose virus was initially associated with AIDS and whence the American HIV denomination is derived.

Between October 1980 and May 1981, the United States Center for Disease Control and Prevention detected an inexplicable increase in incidences of Kaposi Sarcoma and pneumonia caused by the protease *Pneumocystis carinii* in adult homosexual males from New York and California. Similar cases would shortly thereafter be seen among Haitian immigrants.

What could there be in common between the sophisticated, middle-class gay "ghettos" and the teeming, miserable Caribbean immigrants that lived in the shadows of skyscrapers?

Given that AIDS is transmitted through sperm or blood, two suspicions insinuated themselves regarding the disturbing confluence between stylized fops and starving immigrants. The first leaned on the hypothesis of infection through sperm, while the second referred to the international market for blood banks.

The spermatic route revealed the results of reiterated excursions of gays on "vacation" amongst the hypersensualized Haitian machos, whose pride at being exceptionally well-endowed is documented in the novel by Dominican writer Manuel del Cabral, *El Escupido*.[1] He who has a penis the size of an arm would have a "sacred phallus," entitled to more than simply libidinous prerogatives.[2]

If instead of fantasizing about the spermatic circuits of AIDS, the blood transmission of the virus is taken into consideration, the hypotheses become less festive. There, perhaps, exists the possibility that the virus entered the United States from Haiti through these transfusions. Haiti was, then, one of the main providers of human blood for the North American hospital market (a macabre exchange that makes visible how the imperialist literally sucks blood from the continent's poorest country).

Setting aside suspicions about entry routes into the United States, where does AIDS really come from? Assumptions in this regard are even more erratic. There is speculation around an "ecological niche" of AIDS adjacent to Lake Victoria.[3] Haitians residing in Zaire[4] during the 1960s and '70s who have since returned to their homeland could have had a role in the transatlantic propagation of the elusive virus. Other versions springing from the territory of pure science and entering into the battlefield of the Cold War mention Cuban soldiers established in Angola as possible smugglers of the virus. Veteran Angolan combatants could have contaminated those graceful Cuban

1 Manuel del Cabral, *El escupido* (Editorial Quintaria, 1970).

2 In the Portuguese version, Perlongher includes a short sentence after "prerogatives" that does not appear in the Spanish: "According to the first suspicions, American gays traveling to Haiti would have returned to the United States bringing the virus in their luggage."

3 Africa's largest body of water connecting Burundi, Kenya, Rwanda, Tanzania, and Uganda.

4 Zaire is currently known as the Democratic Republic of the Congo.

pájaros (faggots)[5] that, after the mass exodus of 1980, transferred the discomforting "guest" to their *yanki* brothers. The majority of these versions are clearly myths, lacking any supporting technical or scientific data (fig. 3.1).[6]

American and French scientists insist on Africa as the likely cradle of AIDS. But regarding its appearance's supposed antiquity, hypotheses diverge. According to analyses of blood plasma collected in Africa since 1959, the American virologist Andre Nahmias from Atlanta claims that around that time there could have already existed at least one case of AIDS. The French professor Peter Piot from Paris infers from the dissemination of the virus (in Zaire, Congo,[7] the Central African Republic, Rwanda, Zambia, Kenya, Uganda, and Tanzania) that, although the epidemic has deeper roots in Africa than in other continents, it could not predate the 1970s. The explosion in the number of victims occurs between 1979 and 1981, but there were isolated cases reported in African patients in Europe in 1976 and 1977, long before the American outbreak.

AIDS seems to be more widespread in Africa (between five and ten percent of the affected populations registering antibodies) than in Europe (where antibodies are found in less than one percent of the samples). But, in comparison with events in the West, where the main "risk groups" are homosexuals and adherents of "junking" (use of injectable drugs), in Africa AIDS is a heterosexual illness affecting more or less equal proportions of men and women, and ten percent of the children.

These attestations contributed, albeit through cruel expedients, to dismantling the myth of AIDS as a homosexual illness but also served to create others. A doctor from Trinidad, for example, does not dismiss the hypothesis that the Black race is more sensitive to the virus. Additionally, forty percent of North American AIDS patients are Mulattoes or Black, even though

5 In the Portuguese, Perlongher translates it to *bichas*.

6 The Portuguese version comes with a cartoon in between Perlongher's scientific analysis (see next page).

7 Congo is currently known as the Republic of Congo.

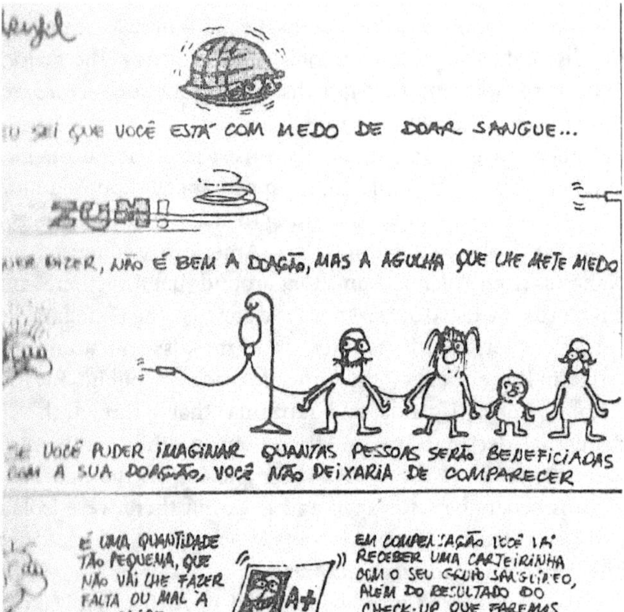
VOCÊ ESTÁ COM MEDO DE DOAR SANGUE...
NÃO É BEM A DOAÇÃO, MAS A AGULHA QUE LHE METE MEDO
VOCÊ PUDER IMAGINAR QUANTAS PESSOAS SERÃO BENEFICIADAS
A SUA DOAÇÃO, VOCÊ NÃO DEIXARIA DE COMPARECER
É UMA QUANTIDADE TÃO PEQUENA, QUE NÃO VAI LHE FAZER FALTA OU MAL À SAÚDE...
A+
RECEBER UMA CARTEIRINHA
ALÉM DO RESULTADO DO CHECK-UP QUE FAREMOS NO SEU SANGUE!
VOCÊ TAMBÉM SABERÁ QUAL A SUA PRESSÃO ARTERIAL, O NÚMERO DE BATIMENTOS DO SEU CORAÇÃO, O SEU PESO E ALTURA CORRETOS!
SERÁ SERVIDO
Obrigado por você!
HEMOCENTRO DO RIO DE JANEIRO
Rua Frei Caneca, 8 - fone 2311290

Fig. 3.1. Cartoon included in the Portuguese version of Perlongher's text. The first three lines from top to bottom read: "I know that you are scared to donate blood"; "That is, it is not really about the donation, but the needle that scares you:" "If you can imagine how many people will benefit from your donation, you would not fail to appear."

campaigns by *Gay Health* were generally led by middle-class whites who confessed to difficulties in entering the racialized "ghettos."

In light of such insinuations, which tend to attribute a sort of "blame" for AIDS to Black populations, the immediate reaction is: Racism! The Haitian government has wielded this argument. An African state prohibited all information related to AIDS, seeing a colonialist conspiracy behind such handwringing. In Bangui, capital of the impoverished Central African Republic, European filmmakers were prohibited from recording footage in hospitals. The special issue of *Le Nouvel Observateur* reads: "The Central African Republic is ashamed of the illness because it reveals customs of which Westerners disapprove."[8]

What could have been those reproachable customs? First of all, promiscuity (including the heterosexual kind). The disorderly growth of African cities after decolonization could have led to a general relaxation of customary mores.

In that context, wherein misery is conjoined with lust—excluding, however, the rigorously clandestine homosexual males, the use of protection is considered an insult. Nor is there a form of convincing contaminated women to stop bearing children.

Moreover, hygienic practices of the developed metropoles are only with difficulty transplanted into zones of extreme poverty. One of the causes of the spread of AIDS rests in the use of unsterilized syringes, which, due to the absence of sanitary conditions, are used with countless patients. As such, African populations suffer from more "curable" illnesses and die from lack of nourishment and technical resources—hospitals in Central Africa even lack X-ray plates.

8 Elisabeth Schemla, "Sida: la tragédie africaine," *Le Nouvel Observateur* 1157 (January 9, 1987), 40. In the French, the quote follows "parce que'elle risque aussi de dissuader les investisseurs européens (because it also risks deterring European investors)."

The Viral Wars Continue

In Africa the medical investment in studying the evolution of AIDS has provided promising, albeit polemic, results. The African hypothesis is based on the discovery of new viruses, named—continuing the struggle over nomenclature—HTLV-IV (by the Americans) and LAV 2 (by the French).

In November of 1986, both the French and the American AIDS teams almost simultaneously announced their findings. Luc Montagnier of the Pasteur Institute delivered the news from Lisbon, where he was participating in a seminar. He collaborated with the French-trained Portuguese researcher María Odette Santos Ferreira, who had the honor of photographing this new virus for the first time. Hours later, alerted by an alleged spy, his rival, Doctor Max Essex, proclaimed from Boston a similar discovery.[9]

The LAV 2 virus was isolated in two male patients from Guinea-Bissau (a former Portuguese colony) and contained genetic similarities with another virus, of animal origin, which often attacks the African green monkey.

The discovery of the HTLV-IV virus, on the other hand, came from a group of Swiss researchers, who isolated it in African patients, among whom the virus' presence did not result in a fatal outcome. Later, it was isolated in three prostitutes from Dakar (Senegal), none of whom were ill. A certain similarity with the virus found in the green monkey tended toward consolidating the hypothesis of a virus transmitted to man by monkeys, although conclusive evidence is still lacking.

Behind the international effort of specialists to gather information about the virus and its origins, mutations, etc., there hides a dance of millions: of credit, of contracts, of prestige, and of interests. "The race for the cure to AIDS promises figures in

9 While Essex was already working on a virus surface protein for blood screening, which is now used for HIV detection, he discovered the first simian immunodeficiency virus and HIV-2, one of the two strands of HIV.

the millions," alerts the magazine *Veja*,[10] under the title "Healthy Business." Even the discrepancy regarding the name of the virus reached the papers. Although the French doctor Luc Montagnier was the first to announce the discovery of a method for cloning (making synthetic copies in the laboratory) the AIDS virus, the corresponding patent was conceded to his rival, Doctor Robert Gallo. In light of this concession, it is estimated that in the coming years Gallo will earn around two hundred million dollars. Naturally, this mass of money works its way through diverse capitalistic operations. Announcing a definite discovery in the field of AIDS, a biotechnological company in California achieved an immediate increase in its share prices.

A Virus Created in a Laboratory?

The suspicion that AIDS was the result of laboratory experiments linked to bacteriological warfare accompanied the saga of the illness like a legendary insignia. This idea was in many places the initial reaction of gays. The homophilic Left of California conjured up the specter of a supposed conspiracy destined to eliminate them.

Outside those circuits the rumor started to unfold in a fabulous way. Accusations came from the Right and the Left, during an ebb in Cold War hostilities. In 1984, in a Seminar on Psychological Warfare in Pretoria, accusations arose against "homosexual partisans of Fidel Castro fighting in a medical warfare unleashed by Cuba and the USSR."[11]

Suspicions cast on North American scientists are a bit more serious. To name a few precedents: the experimental adminis-

10 "Saudável negócio- a corrida da cura da AIDS tem cifras millonárias," *Revista Veja* 898 (November 20, 1985), 132.

11 While the specific seminar couldn't be found, Perlongher is referring to the right-leaning South African National Defense (SANDF) integration of a Psychological Operation (PSYOP) as part of their strategies to counter a network of leftist ideologies. This is key in Perlongher's historical placing of HIV/AIDS in relation to the Cold War and the impending dissolution of the Soviet Union in 1991.

tering of LSD on persons unaware of its application during the 1950s and the macabre experiment performed on (and against) four hundred indigent Black patients suffering from syphilis, given placebos in order to study the pathological effects otherwise eliminated by antibiotics. Some of those patients survived until the age of thirty but ultimately died of syphilis. In 1970, senator Edward Kennedy denounced the administering of radiation treatments, with questionable consent, on a group of 111 cancer patients.

Regarding AIDS, rumors tell of experiences with biological warfare, realized between 1971 and 1978, in a secret laboratory of the North American army at Fort Detrik, Maryland, meant to introduce the swine flu, whose pathologies show similarity with that of AIDS, to Cuba.

Anticipated by Soviet and Hindu tabloids these rumors gained momentum in 1986, when three scientists of certain fame break the same news: The AIDS virus was fabricated in a laboratory, mixing the Visna-Maedi virus found in sheep with the generative agent of leukemia found in cattle, and due to the mishandling of the artificial virus, initially considered inoffensive, it was disseminated. Consequently, those scientists — Seak (England), Streeker (USA), and Segal (Western Berlin) — dismiss the green monkey hypothesis, as it has been in contact with humans for millennia.

The laboratory theory was rejected as ridiculous, and its hypotheses were disproved with indignation. Yet, the polemic remains. Its influence transcends advances in medical science and has immediately political consequences.

Overall, the possibility of AIDS having emerged from a laboratory accident, which would oblige us to reflect on the legitimacy of certain high-risk experimentations done in the name of knowledge, did not unnerve researchers. As such, French scientists, in collaboration with doctors from Zaire, began to experiment on human test subjects with AIDS vaccines and experimental drugs in December of 1986. Questioned by the press, the immunologist Daniel Zagury, in charge of the project, refused to disclose details, taking refuge in scientific confidentiality. Despite the inherent danger vaccines pose to volunteers, the risk may have been worth it. The discovery of an efficient vaccine against AIDS would guarantee a potential market calculated at around one hundred million dollars. [12]

12 Currently thirty-day supplies for HIV retroviral therapy range from $1,500 to $5,000. While insurance policies and health initiatives like the Ryan White HIV/AIDS program through the AIDS Assistance Program (ADAP) facilitate the costs of these therapies in the United Sates, it is estimated that without insurance or without these programs an annual supply ranges between $18,000–$60,000 per person. According to recent HIV/AIDS statistics, approximately 1.2 million people live with the virus with 1 out of 8 not knowing their status. See "U.S. Statistics," *Hiv.gov*, https://www.hiv.gov/hiv-basics/overview/data-and-trends/statistics.

AIDS in Brazil[1]

The illness arrived in Brazil as a fashion statement. While credit is to be given to dermatologist Valeria Petri for detecting, at the end of 1982, the first two Brazilian cases of AIDS (two men, thirty and thirty-two, with Kaposi Sarcoma after traveling to the United States), the death of the fashion stylist Markito began the plague's spectacularized resonance.[2] His agony, meticulously detailed by the mass media, triggered the first wave of local fear.

Initially, it was believed that the diffusion of the illness was restricted to a circuit of the wealthiest of gays, those able to take frenzied getaways to the States. It was, with an ironic tinge, a "chic illness." This bleak trend was not monopolized by mundane spaces, instead expanding rapidly to medical offices. "Illnesses, like everything else, become fashionable," admits Doctor Jean Claude Nahoum (interviewed by the *Médico Moderno* magazine in July of 1985), for whom such a fashion "is not neces-

1 Sources in this section, like in some other parts of the book, come from magazines, journals, newspapers, and headlines that Perlongher was reading and quoting without providing the full citation. Some were able to be retrieved and referenced, others were partially referenced, and some could not be found.

2 Also known as Marcus Vinícius Resende Gonçalves, he was considered one of the first Brazilian victims of AIDS and later died in 1983, while in New York.

sarily an increase of the epidemic's appearance, but its increased incidence in doctors' heads." AIDS, according to him, was not a new disease, but rather a "new systematization of pre-existing elements; in the case of AIDS, this construction was studied initially in homosexuals, insistently looked for among homosexuals, and, naturally, found in homosexuals. From then on, an unequivocal relationship between AIDS and homosexuality was established."[3]

Brazilian homosexuals did not remain insensitive to such an "unequivocal relationship." In July 1983, O Grupo Outra Coisa — Ação Homossexualista (Another Type of Homosexual Action Group),[4] in alliance with San Pablo's Health Center, started to distribute cautionary pamphlets on every corner of San Pablo's slums. The flyer urged gays to be selective, "like you always do," with their sexual partners,[5] and also recommended to not panic. In the case of any suspicion, it recommended they contact the nearest AIDS patient medical service center, which the Sanitary Dermatologist Directive agreed to facilitate under pressure from homosexual activists.

The eruption of AIDS caught Brazilian gays in a paradox. The organic debility of the basically unstructured gay groups (still surviving only on the impetus of the Bahia gay group) coexisted alongside an expansive advertisement of the gay spectacle. The *destape,* the tropical version of *out of the closet* (literally "out of the armoire") of the North American gay, had not favored the bearers of the newly *assumed homosexual* model (one who

3 Source could not be retrieved.

4 The group was founded in 1980 by sexual dissidents of the group SOMOS, a militant group based in São Paulo, Brazil. After having traveled to Brazil in the 1970s, Perlongher exiles himself indefinitely in São Paulo in 1981 where he was given by Teza Aarão a copy of *O bandeirante destiempo: O guia gay de São Paulo* (*The Timeless Pioneer: The Gay Guide to São Paulo*), a publication by Grupo Outra Coisa – Ação Homossexualista.

5 Perlongher uses here and below the French word *partenaire* (partner).

maintains an equal relationship with the assumed homosexual, both without mannerisms).[6]

Transvestites, who had little to do with this program of sexual equality, took advantage of this opening to stage a massive invasion of the avenues of the megapolis. The provocative consecration of the transvestite Roberta Close as "national woman model" could well symbolize a certain erroneous swallowing whole of homosexuality, as suggested by the mass media around 1984. With the appearance of AIDS, these frames would change. The sensual ambivalence of Roberta Close would be substituted for the severe glows of Doña Risoleta, the widow of Tancredo Nieves.[7]

There is, in the AIDS crisis, an aura of restoration. We went too far; guilty, we now pay for the excesses of lust! *A return to monogamy, a turn to the family,* and the definite death of anonymous and impersonal sex....

In the summer of 1985, the death of dramaturg Roberto Galizia — quarantined behind infirmary glass, spending his last days almost blind, dictating poems to his nurse — signals the beginning of a second wave of panic. The rites of agony would, from now on, be rehearsed incessantly in the media.

Television plays a decisive role in making a spectacle of death, standing on the shore of obscenity itself: a scene of two young gay men holding hands lovingly is followed by one of patients eaten away by Kaposi Sarcoma; panoramas of the gay ghettos are followed by martyrdom in a hospital bed. The medical imagery is, in turn, terrorism. During the informational meetings convoked by the recently created Grupo de Apoyo y Prevención del SIDA (GAPA) (Group for the Support and Prevention of AIDS), those in attendance — basically all homosexuals — were bombarded with slides of gnawed glutes and disfigured faces. Later, in 1986,

6 The Portuguese version of *destape* is *desbunde*. It carries a localized archive of dissident sexuality and desire.

7 Risoleta was a central political figure in Brazil. She was married to Tancredo Neves who was elected president after the end of the dictatorship (1964–1985) through the Brazilian Democratic Movement Party, but before taking office in 1985 he died due to diverticulitis.

the painter Darcy Penteado, screaming "medical terrorism!," withdraws from a conference of San Pablo's then Secretary of Municipal Health for exhibiting, on screen, a man deformed by AIDS. Darcy's reaction is not only emotional. According to him, "the problem of AIDS is not the illness itself, rather the paranoia created by the mass media," and denounced how "such media is conspicuously tied to powerful multinational pharmacological schemes that intend to charge egregious amounts for the costs of AIDS; a dishonest medicine, allied to conservative groups, savages, and extremists, pretending to restore old horrors on the back of this new one."[8]

Not all spokespersons of the so-called "risk groups" were so straightforward early on. The reduction of promiscuity and penetration during homoerotic encounters was still bluntly insisted on, even if it meant abstinence: "Between cruising and living, I choose to live," declared the spokesperson of GAPA in May 1985.

Meanwhile, AIDS was escaping from the golden citadel of the *jet set*. Acclimatizing and nationalizing itself, its propagation took on uniquely Brazilian characteristics. Not only were class barriers rapidly delineated (by the end of 1986, ninety-five percent of all AIDS patients came from the popular classes); those of the homosexual slums, where it was initially confined, were gradually weakening. Although contaminated homosexuals still constituted the vast majority of the infected population, the rate of infected "bisexual" men suffered a progressive increase.

This redistribution of pathological quotients becomes worrisome when taking into consideration the differences between the carnivalesque heterogeneity of Brazilian homosexuality and a certain behavioral (and even residential) uniformity implicit in the American gay model, both being derived from different histories.

Indeed, after the harsh repression of McCarthyism during the 1950s, the explosive emergence of *Gay Liberation* after a confrontation between gays and the police in the New York bar

8 "Mecidina e Saúde," *Istoé* (1986): 38–39.

"Stonewall" in 1969 would lead to a certain "territorialization" of North American homosexual populations, who had come out from hiding in the closet with such wild abandon. There were tangible migrations to the major gay ghettos (entire neighborhoods inhabited solely by homosexuals) of New York and California. The city of San Francisco, as the epicenter of hippies and beatniks, became capital of the gay world, a world of closed circles where gays only come into contact with other gays (which could explain the limited dissemination of the illness) but also of real *laboratories of sexual experimentation*, whose repercussions would produce interesting ripples and combinations in neighboring circles. Thus around 1978 it was not infrequent that the routine changes of partners among young Californians included, without drama, a homosexual partner. The new American sexual model did not subsume these versatile lovers under the category of "bisexuals."

This paradigm of sexual identification, which divides individuals according to their amorous object into "homosexuals," "heterosexuals," and "bisexuals" and which reigns in US bedrooms, would be almost literally transplanted to Brazil's much more complex sexual landscape, when the time came to formulate medical and paramedical strategies for combating AIDS. Such a model, which seems to be implicit in the "affirmation of a sexual identity" by some local gay activists, albeit in somewhat diluted forms, has the merit of seeming simple and objective. Unfortunately, a considerable part of the most "popular" reigning homosexual practices "south of the equator" run the risk of falling outside that schema. For example, the term "bisexual" is unheard of in the baroque local nomenclatures. (The diverse homosexual circuit at the heart of São Paulo alone has more than fifty ways of alluding to styles and genders of homosexuality, from the "baby-girl"[9] to the "rent boy."[10]) "Bisexual" would be, when translated into the ghetto's current codes, a type of closeted gay that runs from its established heterosexual family in search of an androgenous adventure. In March 1986, the feminist magazine *Nova* fixated on said topic, writing about "a typical representative" of this disturbing species: "Everaldo, thirty-nine years of age, an executive at an insurance company, has three children and a wife with whom he carries on an enjoyable but sporadic sexual life and never went to a gay[11] bar. He does not know any self-declared gay[12] and does not consider himself one, either. He attends a porn theater close to his office one day a week. There he has casual sex with other men, limiting his stay to no more than thirty minutes" ("quick and raging sex," synthesizes the sentimental monthly).[13]

The inconsistency between the promotion of sexual prevention and actual homosexual practices is not simply rhetorical. Thus, while on the ground in Campinas, the AIDS medical group felt this disjuncture palpably: "What you recommend has nothing do to with the type of sex I practice," complained the suburban homosexual while at the clinic.

---

9 Perlongher utilizes the term *loca-baby* in the Spanish to signal the Southern Cone's localized forms of nonnormative sexualities, which can encompass trans* subjects, transvestites (or travestis), homosexuals, and other gender-nonconforming peoples. In the Portuguese he uses *bicha-baby,* bicha meaning "girl" or "sis," both terms of endearment for gender non-conforming peoples, though *bicha* can also be used as a derogatory term.

10 In the Portuguese, Perlongher uses *michê-gilete* instead of my translation of "rent boy," the first part refers to sex work and the second part to bisexuality. The combined term refers to a bisexual sex worker or sex swinger. In the Spanish, he uses *vuelta y vuelta,* loosely translated as "coming and going" to indicate the oscillation or swinger aspect of sexuality.

11 In English in the Portuguse original.

12 In English in the Portuguse original.

13 Perlongher is referring to the article "Ainda existe vida gay depois da AIDS? As assutadoras mudanças nas relações homossexuais masculinas (Is There Still Gay Life After AIDS? The Frightening Changes in Male Homosexual Relationships)," *Nova: Cosmopolitan,* March 1986.

In the case of Brazil, preventative recommendations directed to homosexuals came together, at first, in a *progressive* strategy aimed at safeguarding, even at the price of self-control, those tenuous human rights acquired by erotic minorities. While "progressive" medicine advocates for certain *reforms* of bodily practices, which diminish the statistical probabilities of the virus's transmission, other less thoughtful sectors advocate more aggressive methods (the type that "ends with the ill to end with the illness").

The urge for greater rigor often goes hand in hand with divine proclamations. Believers from the Asamblea de Dios (Assembly of God) call for exorcisms in the São Paulo ghettos, where they distribute explosive anathemas that call to salvation. The pamphlets tremble with the resonances of inquisitorial regiments that condemned sodomites to burn at the stake. Sodomy was also called — with reason — "the cleric's vice," making clear that everything that touches on such a delicate topic would provoke uneasiness in the Church (exacerbated by the transmission of AIDS among its priests).

Many of the religious contributions concerning the modern plague center on sin and divine punishment. The Jehovah's Witnesses preach that "immorality, an illness of the spirit, has accumulated an abundant set of physical epidemics," just as Jesus has prophesized, and also foretell how in the Kingdom of God "the epidemic of immorality would end." The Iglesia Universal (Universal Church) announces a warlike God: "AIDS is God's slap in the face to homosexuals." For Baptists, it is a "merciful interference" by the Creator: "Wouldn't this be a warning against this abomination (homosexuality), coming from God Almighty?"

The Catholic representatives are far less noisy. The archbishop of Rio de Janeiro, after denouncing how "homosexuality, as sickness or voluntary deviation, looks to revendicate the outsides of normativity," finds a positive side to the plague: "Society's punishments serve as a tool to reawaken the conscience, to censure a reigning immorality, and to return humanity to the paths of God."[14] More level-headed, the assistant bishop of Salvador, while not rejecting the thesis of a "divine wrath," stops short of seeing a positive element in the AIDS crisis: "The AIDS virus could also provoke a positive reaction in relation to the sexual behaviors of all communities: obliging people to evaluate their own sexuality and their *modus vivendi*." At the same time, the archbishop of São Paulo announced the opening of a hospital for those ill with AIDS.

Although less concerned with the capriciousness of divine will, medical protocols, issued in the name of science, are not more reassuring. There were even some that refused, from fear of contamination, to perform an autopsy on victims of AIDS. For Paulo Francis, doctors don't really know much about AIDS: "They talk about viruses. Virus is the most meaningless word in medical mystification, it validates all that doctors don't know."[15] Paranoia extends even to the pharmacists. One of them refused to vaccinate gays, because, if contaminated, "no one at home would want to know the story; everyone would believe I turned queer."[16]

Before the viral nature of AIDS became known, some doctors generously placed the blame and guilt on inmates. One doctor from Bahia attributed AIDS to "an exaggerated consumption of female hormones, a common practice among gays."[17] A colleague from São Paulo added: "AIDS has a preference for the male sex." Around 1984, another Bahian professor, in light of a large quantity of homosexual victims of AIDS, deduced "a pre-

---

14 These words come from the Portuguese, from the Roman Catholic Cardinal Dom Eugênio de Araújo Sales, found in *Revista Veja* which reported that, from 1987 to 1993, thirty-five priests had died of AIDS.

15 This citation is omitted in the Spanish version. It comes from *Folha de S. Paulo: Um journal a serviço do Brasil* 25, no. 20,549 (July 1985). Title of piece and page could not be retrieved.

16 In the Portuguese *virei a mão* means to turn or twist your hand, a gesture of turning gay.

17 In *Revista Veja,* July 1982. Herbert Daniel in "A AIDS é um tigre de papel... higiénico (AIDS is a tiger made out of a hygiene paper)" also cites Perlongher's reference.

disposition possessed only by inverts or that it is acquired in their deviations."

Under multiple nonsensical, contradictory, and imprecise proclamations, the target of this campaign became clear: homosexuals and, more specifically, homosexual promiscuity or "anonymous sex." This type of practice, where two or more subjects make eye contact or simply rub against each other and then, sometimes without exchanging words, become entangled in corporeal frenzy and which is prevalent in homosexual circles is partially derived from the history of segregation and secrecy traditionally imposed on these couplings. Always fleeing persecution, time is lost in florid courtships. But such sensual exuberance among modern gays also fits within the secret tradition of the orgy, which undermines official histories as its subterranean plot.

The vagaries of this aberrant desire can be read in the underground histories of Brazil. The veil of stigma at times forecloses passions that were discretely consummated in the shadows.

During the momentum of the 1970s, and to the rhythm of "coming out," there was some expansion of the unstable threshold of permissiveness for openly homosexual practices. The tenuous liberalization took different routes: diffusion of the influence of gay groups and their representatives; the unveiling[18] of homosexual populations, inhabiting and contesting spaces in certain areas of large cities; and, concomitantly, the proliferation of commercial establishments, nightclubs, bars, saunas, etc., which by consolidating a micromarket of gay consumers contributed to a deepening of class differences blurred by the older, shadowy ways.[19]

In São Paulo, the eruption of AIDS radicalized on a spatial level the progressive emptying of the gay ghetto at the heart of the city. This alteration of territorial density attracted the attention of the police, which took advantage of decreased popula-

18 "Unveiling" is *destape* in the Spanish version while in Brazilian Portuguese it is *desbunde*.

19 Perlongher is pointing to the micropolitical proposed by Gilles Deleuze and Félix Guattari in *A Thousand Plateus: Capitalism and Schizophrenia*, trans. Brian Massumi (University of Minnesota Press, 1987), 208–31.

tions to occupy areas historically won by queers. At a certain, determinate moment, the fervent circulation[20] of gays, faggots, chongos, transvestites, and all those "in between"[21] seemed to have ceased. (At the same time, local secretive spaces, like cinema bathrooms, were reactivated, as if, in face of a moralizing threat, the affected opted for a return to clandestinity.)

Saunas are, appropriately, the most heated point of discussion in the delicate question of AIDS. Paradoxically, they were originally of hygienic origin, and some still function according to the therapeutic model. In the more modern gay saunas, in a true perversion of any hygienic function, the only heat is the heat of sex. They are orgiastic locales with specially darkened lounges for the confusion of sweating bodies. Insofar as sexual athletes find there the conditions required to break all records, one must suppose that, seen from the perspective of the probability of AIDS's propagation, the sauna is a dangerous place.

The proliferation of saunas and brothels for men in São Paulo seemed, upon the eruption of AIDS, uncontrollable. Throughout different neighborhoods, new locations were opened with unfinished structures. Those attending were neighborhood lads accustomed to using the obscurity of the steam for both safe and lascivious acts. Timidly, heterosexual equivalents of these steamy chambers, until then dominated by the business of female prostitution, were liberalized. In a certain distinguished neighborhood, the indiscriminate admission of solitary men and women was allowed.

AIDS came to intervene in this still incipient, processual relaxation of norms. If the preferred target of campaigns was the masculine homosexual, the moralistic offensive also targeted a type of *liberated woman*. Once again, the magazine *Nova* offers a disturbing portrait of such a woman: Sheila, thirty years old,

20 In the Portuguese, Perlongher uses *trottoir* to connote the movement, which is *trotear* in Spanish, associated with animal-like trotting.

21 *Entendidos* is used in the Portuguese to denote the "assumed knowing" of being different. Faggots as *bichas, michês* as *chongos*, and *travestis* as *transvestites* are my translations from the Portuguese version.

"was accustomed to sleeping with different men when she felt like it." She does not show the slightest fear of AIDS, which leaves the reporters worried. The latter launch into paranoic predictions about this evil's eventual development among heterosexuals.

The interest of the masses that this *show* of misinformation appealed to also contained a certain morbid delight. Crude descriptions of the vicissitudes of anal sex, of the depth of penetration, of the rush of oral sex, and of the lethality of kissing invaded families' living rooms, complete with narratives about the promiscuous and their diabolical *performances*. A real cocktail of sex and death, it flirted with the pornographic, without assuming it. But when an openly pornographic film, *I Have AIDS* (1986) by David Cardoso,[22] tried to exploit this interest, it faced threats of boycott and faded out, faced with benches abandoned by regular customers, avid instead for films that satisfied their gasping desires. It seems inherent to the campaign around AIDS that homosexual life be truly visualized.

The strident AIDS campaign in Brazil has had some regrettable consequences. In June 1985, one of the most striking episodes was the expulsion of twenty-four gold miners from the Sierra Pelada, accused of parading cross-dressed through the area. The outcasts, stripped bare (from some they tore hair, eyebrows, and eyelashes), were imprisoned in two trucks with signs that read "Gay Transport," then abandoned on the Trans-Amazonian highway. The incident happened nine days after a medical conference on AIDS. The Federal Police led the operation.

Perhaps such insistence on prevention, given an absence of effective treatments, drove armed men to more vigorous actions. The aggressive assaults against gays in São Paulo may provide an idea of the destructive intersection of medical discourse and its police interpretations. Moreover, the series of shootings directed at transvestites throughout 1986 was attributed, by these same police, to supposed AIDS victims seeking revenge, but ulti-

22 David Cardoso, dir., *Estou com AIDS* (Dacar Produções Cinematográficas, 1986).

mately served only to remove them from the streets using more direct methods than the simple fear of disease. These events are inscribed within the framework of a redoubled violence against erotic dissidents hiding behind the specter of AIDS.

Preoccupied with the illness's advances and unsatisfied with the broad collaboration of organized gay groups, the medical sector begins to propose legislative changes.

It is quite probable that these "new special legislations" have less to do with a grounded fear of the evil's spread among the heterosexual population, than with a certain tendency to transform *prevention* into *repression*.

Perhaps this is not so much about generalized oppression (an optimistic inference based on a certain strategic tendency of police power in Brazil, previously more focused on redistribution and control of territories and their marginal spaces than on a radical extirpation of perverts), than it is about stricter control of suspects and their practices. Patrols of the Brasília ghettos by the military police hunting those susceptible to homoerotic charms indicates how, under the auspices of AIDS, quotidian freedoms such as the right to freedom of movement, are curtailed.

If the preventative measures against AIDS were to evolve from internment of already established cases to the isolation of possible suspects, the shadow of a new type of pogrom (similar to the anti-Semitic persecutions of Central Europe) would lurch, gloomily, into sight. Equally daunting perspectives infer an eventual generalization of testing to the entire population: a subject's blood composition could, in this pessimistic utopia, become an uncontestable criterion for determining the inclusion or exclusion of whomever from any social circle.

Fig. 4.1 (opposing page). AIDS in 1987: The Government of José Sarnay takes A Campaign against AIDS.[23]

23 Sarnay was part of the Democratic Alliance post-dictatorship and ruled from 1985–1990. The Image and caption do not appear in the Spanish

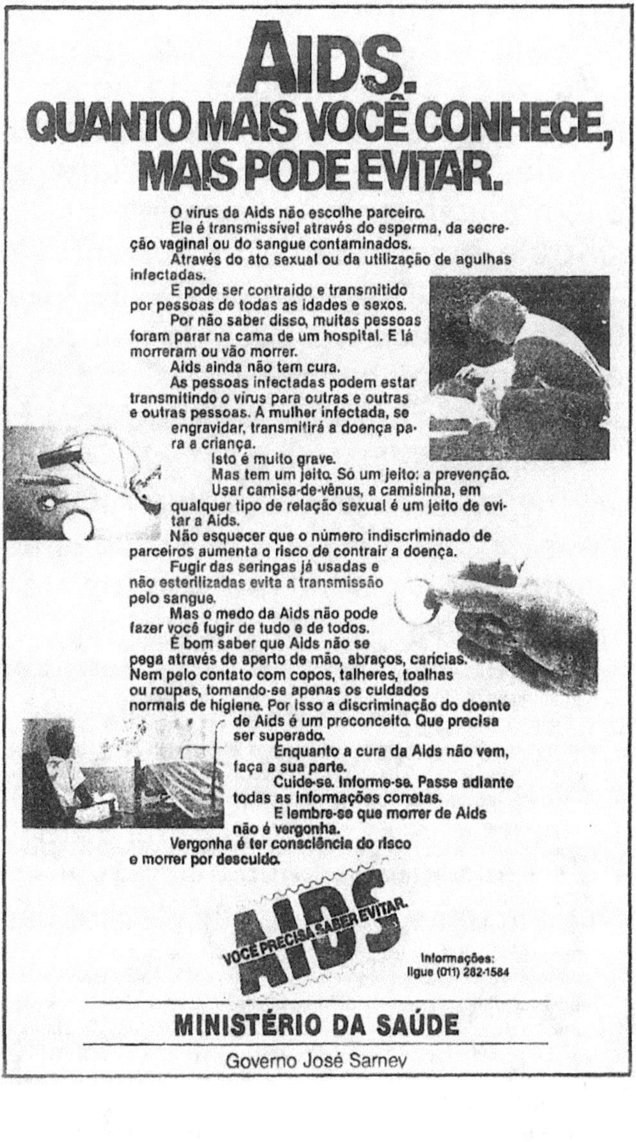
AIDS.
QUANTO MAIS VOCÊ CONHECE, MAIS PODE EVITAR.
O vírus da Aids não escolhe parceiro.
Ele é transmissível através do esperma, da secreção vaginal ou do sangue contaminados.
Através do ato sexual ou da utilização de agulhas infectadas.
E pode ser contraído e transmitido por pessoas de todas as idades e sexos.
Por não saber disso, muitas pessoas foram parar na cama de um hospital. E lá morreram ou vão morrer.
Aids ainda não tem cura.
As pessoas infectadas podem estar transmitindo o vírus para outras e outras e outras pessoas. A mulher infectada, se engravidar, transmitirá a doença para a criança.
Isto é muito grave.
Mas tem um jeito. Só um jeito: a prevenção.
Usar camisa-de-vênus, a camisinha, em qualquer tipo de relação sexual é um jeito de evitar a Aids.
Não esquecer que o número indiscriminado de parceiros aumenta o risco de contrair a doença.
Fugir das seringas já usadas e não esterilizadas evita a transmissão pelo sangue.
Mas o medo da Aids não pode fazer você fugir de tudo e de todos.
É bom saber que Aids não se pega através de aperto de mão, abraços, carícias. Nem pelo contato com copos, talheres, toalhas ou roupas, tomando-se apenas os cuidados normais de higiene. Por isso a discriminação do doente de Aids é um preconceito. Que precisa ser superado.
Enquanto a cura da Aids não vem, faça a sua parte.
Cuide-se. Informe-se. Passe adiante todas as informações corretas.
E lembre-se que morrer de Aids não é vergonha.
Vergonha é ter consciência do risco e morrer por descuido.
AIDS
VOCÊ PRECISA SABER EVITAR.
Informações: ligue (011) 282-1584
MINISTÉRIO DA SAÚDE
Governo José Sarney

version. The lines of the poster read from top to bottom: "AIDS: THE MORE YOU KNOW, THE MORE YOU CAN AVOID. The AIDS virus does not choose a partner. It is transmitted through semen, vaginal secretions, or contaminated blood. Through sexual acts or using infected needles. And it can be contracted and transmitted by people of all ages and sexes. By not knowing this, many people end up in a hospital bed. And there, they die or will die. AIDS still has no dure. Infected people can be transmitting the virus to others, and others to other people. An infected woman, if she becomes pregnant, will transmit the disease to the child. This is very serious. But there is a way. Only one way: prevention. Using a condom in any type of sexual relationship is a way to avoid AIDS. Don't forget that an indiscriminate number of partners increases the risk of contracting the disease. Avoiding used and non-sterilized syringes prevents transmission through blood. But the fear of AIDS cannot make you run away from everything and everyone. It is good to know that AIDS is not caught through handshakes, hugs, caresses. Not by contact with glasses, cutlery, towels, or clothes, or in taking normal hygiene precautions. Therefore, discrimination and prejudice against an AIDS patient needs to be overcome. While a cure for AIDS hasn't come, do your part. Take care of yourself. Inform yourself. Pass on all the correct information. And remember that dying of AIDS is no shame. Shame is to be aware of the risk of dying through neglect."

Homosexuality and Medical Power

The relationship between homosexuality and medicine is manifold. Homosexuality holds a sort of foundational query within medicine, which held the merit of inventing the former's ways of being and doing and defining its territories. In 1869 the Hungarian doctor Benkert[1] coined the term *homosexuality,* substituting the more poetic term *uranism.* These terms replaced, in turn, the old theological dominion over *sodomy.*

This shifting of terms takes part in an operation that is not only rhetorical. Following Michel Foucault (paradoxically a victim of AIDS), from the eighteenth century onward one can situate an ongoing displacement of the problem of the *flesh* (that responded to the celestial hierarchy of sins) toward the axiom of *sexuality.* Such a shift proliferates a vast typology of perverse species of sexual sin where there reigned a less differentiated threat of hellfire.

Some "species" were more fortunate than others. Less is known about the "presbyophiles" or the "dyspaureuniasts" today.[2] Homosexuality, even under the euphemism of "the love

1 Karl Maria Benkert (Kertbeny) (1824–1882) was not a doctor, but rather a writer and human rights activist.

2 Referring to *presbytes* or "old man," a presbyophile refers to someone who likes older men. From the medical term dyspareunia, meaning a difficulty (or pain) in sexual intercourse, a dyspaureuniast is one that enjoys painful

that cannot be named," maintained nonetheless a solid prestige. In principle, it is not that it ceased to be considered a sickness, but that its appropriation has been an object of heated disputes between different branches of knowledge and power: Is it a bio-hormonal deficiency or psychosexual disorder? Convalescent or transgressive? The distinctions between labels are not mutually exclusive; the deployment of these mechanisms can operate simultaneously on bodies in contention.

The proliferation of knowledge and power about sex would also bring forth an increase of perversions, not exactly an undesirable slippage. Such power does not erase pleasure. On the contrary, due to the isolation, intensification, and consolidation of *peripheral sexualities.* previously only a vast amorphous mass, "the relationship between power, sex and pleasure is ramified and multiplied, the body's conduct is penetrated, mediated."[3] From the relationship of power, knowledge, and pleasure emerges a new codification of sex: the *scientia sexualis.*

How do instruments of power penetrate the membranes, the sphincter, the spasmodic undulations, and the iridescence of pleasure? First of all, through the more or less modernized versions of the ancient confessional form: One must tell all about sex. When this information reveals desires, dreams, and fantasies, it is turned over to the psychoanalyst. But the ritual of sexual confession does not, therefore, abandon the asepsis of hospital walls. Rather, present in regular consultation, it intensifies when venereal discomfort enters the waiting room and loses all shame with the slightest suspicion of AIDS.

Beyond confession, the medical arsenal includes less subjective resources, of far more sophisticated technologies. The relationship between patient and doctor then becomes impersonal, anonymous. As compensation, the connection between sickness and medical institution is intensified through deep internal

sex. Later Perlongher would refer to "onanism (self-masturbation)" as a sinful act condemned by the Church for connoting self-inflicting harm.

3 Michel Foucault, *The History of Sexuality,* Vol. 1: *An Introduction,* trans. Robert Hurley (Vintage Books, 1978), 48.

ties and complex instrumentalization that bypass the sufferer's desire or understanding.

The medical gaze is not limited to intervening in the organic but also extends to the regimentation of the subject's life. An example that has nothing to do with AIDS: the creation of maternity programs, along with complimentary material resources and aid (milk, vaccinations, etc.), requiring the beneficiary to follow institutional adjustments of dietary, hygienic, disciplinary, and habitation norms. In sum, a truly disciplinary role that simultaneously adopts a classist position by imposing middle-class medical norms on the beneficiary, to the detriment of their own habits, considered unhealthy.

It is not surprising, therefore, that in the case of AIDS, because the virus can be transmitted sexually, the medical advice enacts a disciplining of sexual practices, especially of homosexuality. It should also come as no surprise that the prophylactic emphasis might decontextualize simple advice and rely on force, in the name of the public good, to make it obligatory. If coercive methods were applied to mothers who resisted participation in pre-partum courses, one could imagine the extent to which the hygienics fervor might go in the case of AIDS patients.

Aside from applying a complex set of common mechanisms to a mass of sicknesses, medical power extracts from AIDS a sort of moral surplus value. This refers back to the long-lasting relationship between medicine and homosexuality.

If the first wave of homosexual liberation was drowned in blood and gas by Nazism, the second propelled the transformation of juridical and forensic norms in First World countries. The removal of homosexuality from the list of mental illnesses by the Association of American Psychologists in 1974 could be considered a symbolic step for contemporary homosexualities in the process of coming out of hiding.

The price for coming out of the shadows was steep. While the homosexual had been transformed into a *species,* endowed with a *personality* centered around its newly discovered sexuality, its predecessor — the *sodomite* — was never more than just someone that practiced anal sex, without the constitution of a "personality" ever being inferred from its "abominable sin."

As it became "tolerated," homosexuality was to be "modeled." Once the so cursed sexuality acceded to the gallery of tolerated enjoyments, homosexuality was expected to show that it could integrate in a disciplined manner to a *broadened* spectrum of *normativity*.[4] This implies, on one hand, a rupture from the marginal masses cohabiting joyously in the darkest corridors of the underground. On the other hand, this separation would also entail their fissure from classical types (faggots, transvestites, and the "top/bottom" folklore), a rupture from "popular homosexualities," occupying golden ghettos of well-educated and artificial gays: such was the expense of visibility.

It cannot be said, however, that the result of gay liberation was exactly chaste. Instead, the residential ghetto, stylishly American, was characterized by an unrestrained promiscuity. It was so explicit that social scientists legitimized that very explicitness. Hence, research in San Francisco in 1970 by sociologists Bell and Weinberg considered that the prototypical "functional" gay was one that had an intense sexual lifestyle and a large amount of partners .[5] Once the role was assumed, it was presumed that no feelings of guilt perturbed its sexual performance.[6] Despite this, the researchers preferred to find in the homosexual couple, long-lasting and sedentary, the paradigm of harmony and total adaptation to the social order.

Homogenization derived from the model gay went quite far in some First World metropolises. All told, the intensification of sexual experience that accompanied homogenization did not cease to provoke intense unease in social circles. The progressive sociologist Castells observed that gays' transgressive perversity was the primary obstacle to the creation of a solid

---

4 In the Portuguese *normalidade ampliada* is used.

5 Perlongher uses here the French word *partenaire* (partner). See, in particular, Alan P. Bell and Martin S Weinberg, *Homosexualities: A Study of Diversity Among Men and Women* (Simon & Schuster, 1978).

6 In English in the original.

alliance between minority groups, which could have provided major political power in the city of San Francisco, where they constitute a significant majority.[7] Indeed, homosexuality was considered *a way of life* and not so much a sexual practice.

Then again, it is worth recognizing that the contemporary transformations of sexual and discursive practices were not only limited to homosexuality. Instead, it forms part of the vast process of the sexual revolution. The unfettered moralization of sickness can be understood as an *a posteriori* consequence of the sexual revolution, where the former is integrated into the latter. Symptoms of a "return to monogamy" are in truth prior to the emergence of AIDS. Repentant feminists, such as Betty Friedan, began to postulate a "return home," arguing that the liberation of women generated, in the end, misery and solitude.[8]

The fact is that the so-called sexual revolution would produce a corporeal excess, made visible not only through the shock of the mass media's spectacle, but also through the expansion of a potent gymnasium industry, among other corporal techniques. Thus, in spite of the radical ideologies of the sexual revolution that advocated for a global interrogation of social values the gradual banalization of permissive sex brought to it a general tedium. Sex lost its rapture, the exciting risk of passion and transgression. In the United States, as a reaction to this programmatic licentiousness, groups started to preach abstinence ("a new form of chastity"). Simultaneously, sophisticated searches for new sensations and singular sexual practices (sadomasochistic and auto-erotic mediums, etc.) were emerging.

An apparatus such as AIDS was only possible beginning from this "ebbing" of the sexual revolution — not the sickness per se,

7 Manuel Castells, "Cultural Identity, Sexual Liberation and Urban Structure: The Gay Community in San Francisco," in *The City and the Grassroots: A Cross-cultural Theory of Urban Social Movements* (University of California Press, 1983), 138–70.

8 Betty Friedan, "The Happy Housewife Heroine," in *The Feminine Mystique* (Dell Publishing Co., 1970), 28–61. In Friedan there is a critique of postwar politics and ideologies that pushed women to return home, creating the domestic confinement or the problem that has no name (11–27).

but the unfettered moralization around it. To achieve the disciplining of the body, one must confess certain scabrous intimacies like penetration, ejaculations inside and outside the anus, and sperm splattering around.[9] If public morality did not allow open discussion of these acts as such, then AIDS would be, like syphilis, a "secret sickness" and perhaps flow from the heroic aura of clandestine adventure.

On the contrary, a campaign like that against AIDS requires as a prerequisite that everything referring to corporality can be said, shown, exhibited, assumed. It is based on this that rulings and diagnoses become possible. In the past the abnormal was excluded from the family and the medical office. Now it can cross that threshold, take a number, and be comforted by consultation.

Once medicine stops considering homosexuality an illness, it focuses on curing or, rather, managing it. The reduction of partners as much as the abandonment of dissolute sexual pleasures tends to impel (at least this is how it seems), rather than the broad repression of homosexual encounters *tout court,* their being placed under medico-institutional control in the sense of a "medicalization" of sex.

How can one not read a certain sensuality in the medical gaze's fixation on the avatars of pleasure? According to Foucault, "The power which thus took charge of sexuality set about contacting bodies, caressing them with its eyes, intensifying areas, electrifying surfaces, dramatizing troubled moments. It wrapped the sexual body in its embrace."[10] With AIDS, the medical embrace will find in the sphincters its point of intervention.

"Anality" comes into play. Science turns its eyes on the anus! The medical machine begins to explore the mucous membranes, points of contact and frictions, microscopic lacerations that testify to an uncontrollable potency. This operation exceeds the secretive locus of the hospital and becomes a spectacle. The objective of this mechanism is to transform the prohibited into

9 "Sperm splattering around" does not appear in the Portuguese version.
10 Foucault, *The History of Sexuality,* 44.

a spectacle, a great show. However, translating the intensity of desires to the normativized schemas of the medical discourse must entail some losses. What before meant enjoyment, in the populous intimacy of orgies, is now projected on a slide as a red flag.

One could ask if the prevailing uncertainties regarding the real efficacy of condoms and spermicides tend to protect, as tribute to conventional morality, a threshold of restrictions. Whatever the case may be, the introduction of a thin latex film between lascivious organs could acquire a symbolic value beyond the therapeutic: an inscription that details, in the fluid whirlwind, the clear presence of the law.

The apparatus of AIDS does not seem to be directed (at least from the progressive perspective) so much at the elimination of homosexual acts, as at the control and redistribution of perverse bodies, aiming to make of the homosexual an aseptic and regulated figure, a sort of perverse statue in the national park. Why exactly, then, is the homosexual the center of this problematic?

If homosexuals are, in some way, medical "creatures," could the appearance of AIDS serve to reintegrate the disobedient back to the flock? Beyond this speculation, it suggests that the "gay way of life" could constitute an avant-garde experiment in creating ever more individualistic models of subjectivation. This means that certain characteristics of gay life — solitude, rootlessness, tearing away from kinship networks, etc. — would become functional or end up being emulated by sections of society that are not necessarily homosexual. If that were the case, it would be necessary to "disinfect" the homosexual so that it would incarnate, without danger or displacements, a certain "way of life" dissociated from the socially undesirable promiscuity. A desexualization of homosexuality?

Solitary Hearts

The programmatic approach to AIDS indicates a shift at the very level of bodily unions. The shift in sexual habits entails a fundamental shift at the heart of the masculine homosexual relationship, which would cease to be centered on the sphincter (that is, on anal penetration) and would come to be centered on masturbation, mutual in the best of cases.

This transformation is now justified by a weighty sanitary reasoning. Nevertheless, in the imposition of the *gay model* there were warning signs regarding slippages on the axis of pleasurable intensities. At the end of the 1970s, specialized researchers observed that within North American homosexuals, sexual acts such as fellatio, mutual masturbation, and rubbing tended to predominate over penetration. However, the latter practice maintained great prestige among Puerto Rican and lower-class homosexuals.

It is revealing that the logic of AIDS should approximate the "Anglo-Saxon" homosexual model, triggering a re-education of more "Latino" forms as allegedly "backward." The conviction with which this operation was carried out explodes when it attributes the delay of a considerable part of affected populations in changing their traditional ways of relating to "misinformation." It is quite probable that there really is a dose of unawareness. However, a reluctance to adopt "healthy" practices could represent to a certain extent a form of "resistant desire" embedded in a history of corporal pleasures.

But going back to masturbation, it is curious that now it is recommended as an alternative when, in previous decades, it was considered the source of various ills and psychosomatic deviations. In light of these recommendations, an innovative practice has emerged in the United States: *phone sex*. The client contacts a specialized agency to select a voice (effeminate or strong, delicate or coarse) that will, depending on the tone, regulate the manipulation of spasms.

Thus, as it becomes regulated, perversion becomes distant and isolated. Perhaps this "receiver sex" indicates a likely culmination of the politics of sexual identity: sex shifts from being a relationship between bodies to a relationship with one's own body. Limited to individualistic monads, one can barely choose their own fantasy in a market of mere artifice.

Against these odds, sectors of the Church were not able to absorb an autoerotic legitimacy. In the planning of the most recent AIDS campaign, they pulled verses from the Bible that condemn masturbation.

The Medicalization of Life

Without needing to dwell on Bible verses, medicine is the main protagonist of the AIDS crisis. Thanks to the echo chamber of the mass media, AIDS as an event has expanded medicine's influence and power without precedent. The masses, obsessed with health and desperate to delegate away their daily ghosts, are pleased by its repetitive and sonorous discourse. Part of a global program to *"medicalize" life*—which, in the last instance, would itself be a "sickness"—medicine confiscates and appropriates death by providing technocratic explanations for ancient fears and subtly selling an illusion of immortality. The medical institution is therefore positioned to legitimize its moral jurisdiction, that is, the power to establish, in the name of wellness, rules of existence.

One senses day to day the consequences of this gradual "medicalization." Certain pivotal life rituals are shifted from the domestic sphere to the confinements of the hospital. Under a suspicious clinical eye that watches over our vital processes, we are born, we breed, we suffer, and we die in modern sanitary temples.

There is no longer a personal relationship with death. The ancient ceremonies of the dying saying farewell from their bed, surrounded by friends and kin, has gone extinct. Dying has become a mere technical phenomenon marked by a hospital unit interrupting life support at a determinant moment. There are the "exemplary patients" that endlessly follow the orders of clinical experimentations and the "unexemplary patients" that resist them. Among victims of AIDS, Rock Hudson would be, for example, the exemplary patient (surrounded by a group of assistants, he faithfully followed all instructions). Designer Markito, however, would be an unexemplary patient, having abandoned treatment after realizing there was nothing else to be done.[11]

Worse yet is that, come the hour of death, it becomes difficult to contain the multiplying interventions and experiments of the medical machine, making for a crueler agony and a more painful death. President Tancredo Neve's sad, prolonged affliction is still fresh in memory, going through and subjected to medical paraphernalia.[12] The terrible thing is that his macabre end might be all of ours.

Even when these spectacular interventions might contribute to advancing knowledge, they do not seem to save as many lives as they publicize. A large part of the diminishing mortality rates in the West is due not to the progress of medical science but to the general betterment of sanitary, dietary, and living conditions. It is not enough to discover a vaccine against a determined pathology if the living environment continues to be gruesome. Mortality produced by pollution and unsanitary labor is far more dangerous. Even as they constantly speak in the name of life, in the current socioeconomic system doctors can become administrators of capitalist deaths.

In the political debate around AIDS, medical discourse seems to consider all bodies and organs as completely regulatable objects. Hence, it confronts an insurmountable resistance: desire. Medicine cannot encapsulate desire since, as it escapes all modifications, desire follows an impulse that is neither rational nor formal. On the other hand, hygienic norms do

11 In the Brazilian context, mass media played a large role in constructing HIV as an epidemic linked to scandalous acts and confessions rather than as a real threat to all Brazilians. The proliferation of this construction can be seen in celebrities such as prominent Brazilian designer Markito or US citizen Rock Hudson who were affected by the virus but contributed to the creation of a public image tying sexual perversion, entertainment, and scandal to the spread of AIDS. See Patrick Larvie, "Nation, Science, and Sex: AIDS and the New Brazilian Sexuality," in *Disease in the History of Modern Latin America*, ed. Diego Armus (Duke University Press, 2003), 290–314.

12 Tancredo Neve was a Brazilian politician who had won the presidential elections but suddenly died from cancer a day before taking office.

not emerge from what is pleasing or enjoyable but from frigid technical analyses. Not being able to regulate desire, medicine excludes it by leaving it outside the field of the "real," assuming of course that, according to prophylactic conventions, existential trajectories could be regimented, jeopardizing, however, the flows of arousal, passions, and intensities.

Medicine's aversion to desire extends to the use of drugs, which are only to be provided to a patient as long as there is no suspicion that the patient finds some sort of enjoyment in them. Additionally, free distribution of syringes has been suggested for users of injectable drugs in order to decrease the transmission of AIDS through blood. Though reasonable, such a measure may mean opening the floodgates to certain stigmatized, "unhealthy," and uncontrollable avenues.

The Order of Death in the Disorder of Bodies

Aside from a therapeutic value, the distribution of recommendations regarding AIDS, that divides sexual encounters into advisable or unadvisable depending on risk level, seems to speak of a certain *regime of bodies*. A close examination of their nature perceives a determinate *organization of organs*, a functional hierarchy of the organs: the mouth to eat, the ass to shit, the penis for the vagina, etc. Alternative uses of the body tend to be considered unnecessary. Anal sex especially (recall São Paulo's gay slogan at its contestatory apogee: "Anal sex topples capitalism"[1]) is the target of medico-journalistic operations related to AIDS. While some commentators recognize that an excess of sensationalism conceals far more serious illnesses (such as the epidemic of Alzheimer's), they still consider AIDS to be "mostly avoidable." Such assumptions rest on a widely held belief: Anal sex, which does not (re)produce anything, would be, in contrast to vaginal sex, unnecessary, an aberration or deviance unrelated to "natural" virtues and therefore only to vice's misfortunes.

1 Famous slogan by the Brazilian militant group SOMOS, members that included William Santos and Olavo do Carvalho.

Sodomy constitutes a strong site of prohibitions within Judeo-Christianity, in particular in the Middle Ages.[2] Certainly, these arguments have changed. If the Inquisition had attempted to avoid the spilling of sperm destined only for procreation and the benefit of God's earthly figureheads, contemporary stances on sodomy manifest via an appeal to medical knowledges, forms of prescription destined to prolong the supervision of the patients in their care (practically the entire population).

Sodomy and de Sade

In the work of Marquis de Sade anal sex is charged with subversive connotations. Ritualized as a discourse that rhythmically patterns orgiastic aberrations, sodomy was revered as an exaltation *contra natura* that defied—just like kissing the devil's ass—sexophobia and proclaimed the death of both the king and the divine. But the fascinations of sodomy are not exhausted in this symbolic deicide. *Philosophy in the Bedroom's* Dolmancé had already privileged lust and its enjoyments:

> [A]fter having mused for an instant upon the splendid prospect of a ready and beckoning ass, after having patted it, slapped it a bit, handled it, sometimes after having beaten or whipped it, pinched and bitten it, the rake moistens with his mouth the pretty little hole he is about to perforate, and prepares his entry with the tip of his tongue; in similar wise, he wets his engine with saliva, or with pomade, and gently presents it to the aperture he intends to pierce; he guides it with one hand, with the other he lays wide open the checks of his delight; immediately he feels his member penetrate, he must thrust energetically, taking all due care not to give ground; then it is, occasionally, the woman suffers, if she is new, or young; but, totally heedless of the pangs which are soon to change into pleasures, the fucker must be lively and

2 Second fragment from this sentence was excluded from the Spanish version, but appears in the Portuguese.

> drive his engine ahead, inch by inch, gradually, but with determination, 'till at last he is arrived at his objective, till, that is to say, his device's hairs precisely rub the anal rim of the embuggered party. Then may he give free rein to himself; all the thorns are plucked from out his path, there remain roses only there. To complete the metamorphosis into pleasures of what distresses his object still experiences, if it be a boy, let him seize his prick and frig it; let him twiddle her clitoris, if 'tis a girl; the titillations of the pleasure he will cause to be born will in turn work a prodigious contraction in the patient's anus, and will double the delight of the agent who, overwhelmed with comfort, will soon dart, to the very depths of the ass of his delight, a sperm quite as abundant as thick, thus determined by so many lubricious details.[3]

The Sadean libertine prefers youngsters and the voluptuousness of passivity that unleashes a certain type of "becoming a woman," since "it is delicious to fake being a whore, giving in to a man as if we were women, calling that man our lover, confessing being their lovers." [4]

Beyond these predilections, it seems that the supposed avoidability of "anality" could only be proposed from a "functional" perspective, purely biological and normative. It is not that perverse practices are anchored in the lack of needs, but in excessive pleasures of desire. From an intensive point of view, the pleasures of sodomy, according to Sade, are almost irresistible.

Nomadic Sex

Another problem is the question of promiscuity, orgies, and *nomadic sex.* A certain psycho-medical perspective assumes that erotic bodies universally aspire to a stable, loving relationship. However, nomadic sex is not a manifestation of lack or

3 Marquis de Sade, *Philosophy in the Bedroom,* trans. Richard Seaer and Austryn Wainhouse (Publisher Group West, 1795), 38.

4 Dolmancé in ibid., 51

fruit of lacking stable love, but a will to desiring affirmation that would weave through all these dense and dangerous paths.

The rise of AIDS unleashes an apparatus that attempts to "fix" these nomadic sexualities to promoted "conjugalization." Here we glimpse again the "incomprehension" of medical optics: If it is already difficult to accept the erotization of some organs to the detriment of others with a specific physiological "function," it would be even less likely to understand certain orgiastic or nomadic practices that try to do with a great number of partners[5] what could be done, from a technical perspective, with only one. Medical morality clashes with the combinations of interconnected bodies.

Intensive lines of flight

Wrapped up in a network of social encounters, bodies create intensities. Affects and repulsions between bodies, their sensations, are in themselves intensive. They modulate according to thresholds of intensities, whose production overturns and traverses the bodies, bringing to its extremes or even subverting the organism's physiological organization. At that point, strong searches for *intensity*, for *sensorial ecstasy*, can tense the body until the limit of its resistance, until the threshold of death and disintegration.

These desires tend to excess, disproportion, a line of flight.[6] The paths are endless. An extreme search for intensity can follow the paths of orgies, of radical and systematic perversion, even the extenuation and apathetic repetition of gestures. An always limitrophe line of flight, it is capable of stepping to the edge of destruction and self-destruction's abysses, unchaining a *passion of abolition*.

Both the pervert that wanders in danger's wastelands or the drug user that insists on exacerbating an impossible, frenetic

5 Perlongher uses here and below the French word *partenaire* (partner).
6 Félix Guattari and Suely Rolnik, *Molecular Revolution in Brazil*, trans. Karel Clapshow and Brian Holmes (MIT Press, 2008), 145.

vertigo are submerging themselves in the quicksand where the intensification of desire brushes up onto death. However, this insatiable search is not strictly suicidal, although suicide might appear, as an accident or temptation, in its meandering complexity. This search for intensity is essentially affirmative. It affirms life, tensing it and tensing the body, traveling through the experience of its limits. This experience of radical defiance that, in its intensive exploration, hints at passing through the thresholds of creation and sensation, points to, in the last instance, the mutation of existence, taking the human subject for a traveler between points of flight and rupture. These species of travel cannot be boxed in by the rigid frames of a supposed "rationality." Nor does it integrate itself to the preestablished schemas of a padded and routine existence.

A medical perspective does not tend to take into account these labyrinthine forms of desire but, instead, is based on a linear scheme. From the point of view of "medicalization," life is not apprehended in its *intensive* sense, but only in its *extensive* sense. More important is the statistical frigidity of per capita life expectancy, over and above the richness and quality of lived experiences. Norms will be elaborated, then, in an attempt to prolong the abstract time of life while omitting the singular intensity with which each life is lived. Fear of death invades and confiscates life, restricting expansive potentialities, neutralizing intensities.

Death and Desire

Homosexuality has been traditionally linked to death. As a pejorative imposed on North American homosexuals, the term *faggot* (literally a "bundle of twigs"), it has been said, descends from the timber used to roast sodomites and heretics at the stake. Taken as myth, such a story reinforces an inextricable entanglement of homosexuality and murder, predominant in

Jean Genet's novels, specifically *Querrelle de Brest.*[7] These scenes, concretized as homosexuals, become objects of continuous robberies, extorsions, beatings, and various other crimes (according to the Bahía Gay Group's reports, in two years more than fifty have been murdered), a ceremony of terror that is, at times, part of the game.

AIDS introduces a clinical turn to this sinister relationship. *In a sort of astonishing complicity, morality is conjoined with the pathological.* Without downplaying the real dangers AIDS represents, the weaponization of its lethality to regulate and to torment the perverse must be avoided. To consider AIDS an "avoidable" evil, fruit of excesses we could do without, implies negating, to better domesticate, the force of desire that drives someone to socially "undesirable" relationships. Does not the old conservative illusion of the "avoidability" of homosexuality itself lurk behind the argument that sodomy is "avoidable"?

Perhaps this apparatus hides an intent to lessen the provocative lust of the *locas*[8] by reducing outings and "dissident" sexual experiences through an array of more or less conjugal narrativizing standards. These parameters exclude the promiscuous, the marginalized and transvestites, and eventually liberated women, libertine men, and so on. Hence, in order to escape the diatribe accusing them of being "infectious agents," certain gays would attempt to "clean up their image," constituting themselves as parodic defenders of a nonviolent but emulative normativity. Through a politics of "reform," "dignity," and "homosexual identity," homosexuality paradoxically desexualizes itself by abstaining from the sodomitic delights celebrated by de Sade. In this sense, a large portion of the American gay movement has diluted its contestatory character in order to rearticulate itself as a paramedic organization for public health.

---

7 Written in 1945 and published anonymously in 1947, it appeared officially under Genet's name in 1953. Jean Genet, *Querrelle* (Grove Press, 1974).

8 *Locas* is a South American term for what could be known in North America as queer, faggot, or transvestite. In the Portuguese, *bichas-loucas* is used.

Would it be, perhaps, necessary to conceive a *different form of sexual politics* that does not misrecognize a multiplicity of erotic desires, nor attempt to pedagogically discipline the pleasurable of the perverse? This is about *distributing the best possible information* while simultaneously guaranteeing a right to decide on one's own life and body, already demanded by Engels.[9]

Life is not simply measured, as the medical institutions would have it, in terms of survival's (or agony's) prolongment, but also in the intensity of enjoyment.[10] We must not renege on the desiring dimension of life, if life is what we want to save.

Lastly, the apparatus of AIDS fits into a generalized rightward turn in the West. The American Right would, in large part, attempt to contain a dissolution of morality that it commercialized but which so concerned the Papacy. This articulation of reactionary forces led libertarian philosopher Félix Guattari to say that if AIDS did not exist, they would have had to invent it: "Taken over by reactionary and carnivalesque conservatism, there seems to be a certain type of celebration of death in relation to sickness that develops an obsessive politics of homosexual repression."[11] On top of the AIDS panic will also be the threats of death that already hangs on humanity: hunger, pollution, war, etc., all far more "avoidable" than sodomy.

There is, however, a real risk for threatened populations, one that should not at all be underestimated. It has to do, perhaps, with an unstable compromise between enjoyment and risk, subjected to the oscillations of desire. The assertion that desire should not be lived with guilt or with a bad conscious—as a hysteric hygienics would like—but with contentment. How paradoxical it would be if the fear of death made us lose our enjoyment of life.

---

9 These last four words are omitted in the Spanish, but appear in the Portuguse. It is also the first time Perlongher makes reference to theorist Friedrich Engels.

10 In Portuguese and in Spanish it is *gozo* or *goce*, respectively, gesturing also to the pleasure principle or *jouissance*.

11 Although this sentence is in quotation marks, in the Portuguese it is also italicized, gesturing to a kind of paraphrase of Guattari.

Epilogue

Gabriel Giorgi

It is indeed suggestive that the English translation of *El fantasma del SIDA* by Néstor Perlongher comes right after the publication of Judith Butler's *Who Is Afraid of Gender?* (2024),[1] a book centered on what Butler calls the "phantasm of gender" mobilized by the far right across the globe, a phantasm that brings together and juxtaposes an expanded agenda of violence not only against feminist and LGBTIQ+ movements but also against other precarized communities. Perlongher had identified something similar forty years ago around AIDS, when the battleground was the health system at the very beginning of the neoliberal era. In his book, AIDS becomes *el fantasma del SIDA,* aptly translated by Jorge Sánchez Cruz as "the specter of AIDS." From AIDS to "gender ideology"—as the new rabid conservatives put it—, between South and North, in an increasingly globalized world shaping our historical experience in the last decades, phantasms and specters have become tools of world-making designs against queer lives. From *el fantasma del SIDA* to the phantasm of gender: the history of sexual and gender dissidence, which is fundamentally a history of material embodiments, of practices with and of the body, is always punctuated by these spectral figurations coming out from fear, hate, and the nightmarish

1 Judith Butler, *Who Is Afraid of Gender?* (Farrar, Straus and Giroux, 2024).

vision of a world that, without queer people, without feminists, without transgender people, will finally be ordered, transparent, and legible.

Ordered, transparent, and legible for whom, by whom? For those who are not able to deal with the challenges and the possibilities of desire, and who turn their impossibilities into a form of politics.

Perlongher had a great deal of experience with this kind of people. He was a poet and an activist since the early 1970s, when Argentina, after the victory of Peronist left-wing party in 1973 and the emancipatory energy liberated in that process, was heading toward the worst civil massacre in its history with the reactionary military dictatorship from 1976–1983. Perlongher had participated actively in the formation of the Frente de Liberación Homosexual (Homosexual Liberation Front) or FLH, one of the first queer organizations in Latin America, and started to publish essays and poems in the journal/fanzine *Nuestro Mundo,* a very early publication fighting for sexual liberation, before the censorship of the dictatorship fell upon Argentine public life. By the end of the 1970s, Perlongher exiled himself in São Paulo, Brazil, where he produced much of his work before he died in the early 1990s due to complications of AIDS. *El fantasma del SIDA* from 1988 was his intervention against what he saw as an increased medicalization and disciplining of queer bodies as an effect of the management of the AIDS pandemic.

Perhaps one of the main marks left by Perlongher's writing is the explosion of the feminine in language, *la lengua de las locas* in the precise formula coined by Cecilia Palmeiro: the language of the faggots, of the *marica,* of a femininity out-of-norm, challenging and exceeding the frames of recognizable femininity.[2] The neobaroque as literary style, renamed by Perlongher as *neobarroso* to evoque the muddy shores of the Rio de la Plata, is

2 Cecilia Palmeiro and Mariano López Seoane, "La lengua de las locas," *El lugar sin límites: Revista de estudios y políticas de género* 3, no. 5 (2021): 186–92.

the style of this explosion of the feminine: the verbal excess, the feast of language, the opacity as a strategy against the norm.

This labor of the feminine in language is inseparable from one main figure in Perlongher's queer laboratory of the literary and the political: the *loca,* a figure that can be distantly translated as "faggot" but that retains more explicitly its ties with femininity — *loca* is, after all, a mad woman and also a woman with a very active sexual life outside marriage.[3] This articulation between madness and sexuality at the intersection of gender is what Perlongher mobilizes as a cornerstone from where to think and to perform queerness precisely from the meanings, memories, and challenges embedded in Argentina's culture and language. Paradigmatically, the figure of Eva Perón — the "corpse of the nation," in Perlongher's words — is also a laboratory for this explosion of a queer femininity in his literature and his politics.

As Perlongher elaborates it, the *loca* is a nonidentitarian figure, one that eludes the grammars of identity and the immediate readability of bodies. The *loca* moves between the feminine and the masculine, between the rational and the irrational (it is, after all, the madwoman), between performative and medical vocabularies, more than between recognizable identities. She also attracts social violence and sheds light on the political threshold between the living and the dead, as in Perlongher's classic essay "Matan a una marica" ("A Faggot Is Murdered") where he reads the map of social violence upon the body of a *loca* murdered in the streets. The figure of the *loca* reasserts the powers of the micropolitical, the molecular, the traffic of affects that take place below the recognizable identities, opening the possibility of an excess that can also be strategic and pragmatic in shifting social and political environments.

Perlongher is also a cartographer of the urban peripheries. In his poetry as well as in his essays, queerness is always a *cartografía deseante* (desiring cartography) in which the city is mapped in relation to cruising trajectories that are also an inter-

3 Cecilia Palmeiro, "Ni una menos: Las lenguas locas del grito colectivo a la marea global," *Cuadernos de Literatura* 23, no. 46 (2019): 177–95.

rogation between body and urban life, and between forms of being with others that defy the normalizing design of the city and open new forms of territoriality that emerge from queer life. Against the mechanism of privatization that the emerging neoliberalism will only reinforce to the paroxysmal violence of our days (and Perlongher saw AIDS as a tool for that normalizing goal of the emerging form of domination), his writing will always pursue the life in the streets, in the parks, in the very pockets outside the privatized life where another city and therefore another way of being could come into existence, even if ephemerally.

The publication of *The Specter of AIDS* brings to the fore a much-needed discussion about the 1980s as a direct precursor to the present. Our talks about precarity and precarization, about body politics, about temporalities beyond the grammar of progress and about the very vulnerability of bodies and territories delve into the experimentations and reckonings rooted in the '80s. Perlongher is a key name of this echo that connect that decade with our present. Having this book in English makes it possible, for instance, to create a more productive dialogue between Perlongher's work as writer and activist and the work by David Wojnarowicz, the activist, writer, and artist that became one of the key figures in Act Up. A dialogue of this nature will offer us a hemispheric view of the ways in which the notion of literature and of culture at large was challenged by the new weight of sexual dissidence inseparable from the awareness of the ways in which AIDS became a form of precarization of life at the very dawn of neoliberalism, North and South. The precarious lives that we discuss today as the face of neoliberal policies were epitomized in the HIV lives that these two figures inscribed in our literary and visual archives. They did so by turning the precarious body into a voice of rage, a voice of action, into potency. Wojnarowicz's most known image is perhaps that of his jacket, during a demonstration by Act Up, that reads, "If I die of AIDS, forget burial, just drop my body at the stairs of the FDA." This is also a central force in Perlongher's writing in general, particularly in *El fantasma del SIDA*: the ability to challenge the forces of death by making visible the *political nature of death* in the management of the pandemic. A dialogue between Perlongher and Wojnarowicz could be, in this sense, a true laboratory of the present, one that necessarily takes place between English and Spanish and under a cultural cartography that takes seriously the hemispheric nature of the historical processes that takes us to the present, now in the inflection of the neofascist agenda.

In fact, Paul Preciado argues that our contemporary historical experience is carved upon the epistemic and political shift modeled by the AIDS pandemic, that the COVID-19 pandemic only expanded to a planetary scale.[4] The centrality of immunity and immunization as a cornerstone of medical, political, subjective, and technological vocabularies is just one indication of the ways in which our experience, our bodies, and our thinking are designed by the centrality of virus and virality. Perlongher's early intervention in this discussion will situate the impact of *el fantasma del SIDA* as a disruption within the collective and public circulation of desire. As he writes in the opening of the book, the specter of AIDS is "haunting the streets." He does so within a vaster literary and conceptual take on the disputes shaping the last decades of the twentieth century, that of the ambivalences of desire at the inflection of new, more intense modeling of subjectivities and bodies. At this historical inflection when queer bodies are once again a target of new dreams of sexual and social cleansing, when the "specter of gender," in Butler's formula, articulates new brutal wars on sexual and gender dissidence, the archives of the struggles around AIDS are more relevant than ever. The publication of *El fantasma del SIDA* in English is a decisive and urgent tool for these battles at the heart of the present.

---

4 Paul Preciado, *Dysphoria mundi: El sonido del mundo derrumbándose* (Anagrama, 2022).

Bibliographies

Translator's Bibliography

Baigorria, Osvaldo. "El espacio de la orgía: Una conversación con Néstor Perlongher." *Suplemento* 17 (1985): 4–6.

Bell, Alan P., and Martin S. Weinberg. *Homosexualities: A Study of Diversity Among Men and Women*. Simon & Schuster, 1978.

Ben, Pablo, and Santiago Joaquin Insausti. "Dictatorial Rule and Sexual Politics in Argentina: The Case of the Frente de Liberación Homosexual, 1967–1976." *Hispanic American Historical Review* 97, no. 2 (2017): 297–325. DOI: 10.1215/00182168-3824077.

Butler, Judith. *Who Is Afraid of Gender?* Farrar, Straus and Giroux, 2024.

Castells, Manuel. "Cultural Identity, Sexual Liberation and Urban Structure: The Gay Community in San Francisco." In *The City and the Grassroots: A Cross-cultural Theory of Urban Social Movements*. University of California Press, 1983.

Daniel, Herbert. "A AIDS é um tigre de papel… higiénico." In *AIDS: A Tercera Epidemia: Ensaios e Tentativas*, edited by Herbert Daniel and Richard Parker. ABIA, 2018.

Deleuze, Gilles, and Félix Guattari. *A Thousand Plateaus: Capitalism and Schizophrenia.* Translated by Brian Massumi. University of Minnesota Press, 1987.
Derrida, Jacques. *Of Grammatology.* Translated by Gayatri Chakravorty Spivak. Johns Hopkins University Press, 1997.
"DHS Responds: Coronavirus (COVID-19)." *Department of Homeland Security.* https://www.dhs.gov/archive/coronavirus.
Guattari, Félix, and Suely Rolnik. *Micropolítica: Cartografías del deseo.* Translated by Florencia Gómez. Traficantes de Sueño, 2006.
———. *Micropolítica: Cartografias do desejo.* Vozes, 1986.
———. *Molecular Revolution in Brazil.* Translated by Karel Clapshow and Brian Holmes. MIT Press, 2008.
Engels, Friedrich, and Karl Marx. *Manifesto of the Communist Party.* New York Labor News, 1888.
Foucault. Michel. *The History of Sexuality.* Vol. 1: *An Introduction.* Translated by Robert Hurley. Vintage Books, 1978.
Larvie, Patrick. "Nation, Science, and Sex: AIDS and the New Brazilian Sexuality." In *Disease in the History of Modern Latin America: From Malaria to AIDS,* edited by Diego Armus. Duke University Press, 2003. DOI: 10.1215/9780822384342-012.
Lemebel, Pedro. *Loco afán: Crónicas de sidario.* Editorial Anagrama, 1986.
Muñoz, José Esteban. *Disidentifications: Queers of Color and the Performance of Politics.* University of Minnesota Press, 1999.
Palmeiro, Cecilia. *Desbunde y felicidad: De la cartonera a Perlongher.* Título, 2011.
———. "El deseo como negocio." *Apuntes CECYP* 16, no. 23 (2013): 173–79.
———. "Ni una menos: Las lenguas locas del grito colectivo a la marea global." *Cuadernos de Literatura* 23, no. 46 (2019): 177–95. DOI: 10.11144/Javeriana.cl23-46.nlgm.

Palmeiro, Cecilia, and Mariano López Seoane. "La lengua de las locas." *El lugar sin límites: Revista de estudios y políticas de género* 3, no. 5 (2021): 186–92.

Perlongher, Néstor. *Caribe transplatino: Poesía neobarroca cubana y rioplatense.* Iluminaras, 1991.

———. *Correspondencia.* Edited by Cecilia Palmeiro. Mansalva, 2016.

———. "Devenires minoritarios." In *El lenguaje libertario.* Vol. 2, edited by Christian Ferrer. Nordam, 1991.

———. "Disciplinar os poros e as paixões." *Lua Nova: Revista de Cultura e Política* 2, no. 3 (1985): 35–37. DOI: 10.1590/S0102-64451985000400007.

———. *El fantasma del SIDA.* Puntosur, 1988.

———. "El orden de los cuerpos." *Folha de São Paulo* (1987): n.p.

———. "Los devenires minoritarios." *Revista de Crítica Cultural* 4 (1991): 13–18.

———. "Minoritarian Becomings," translated by Cristel M. Jusino Díaz. *E-misférica* 10, no. 2 (2013): n.p.

———. *O négocio do michê: Prostituição viril em São Paulo.* Editorial Brasiliense, 1987.

———. *O que é AIDS.* Editora Brasiliense, 1987.

———. *Plebeian Prose.* Translated by Frances Riddle. Polity, 2019.

———. *Prosa plebeya.* Edited by Osvaldo Baigorria and Christian Ferrer. Colihue, 1997.

Preciado, Paul. *Dysphoria mundi: El sonido del mundo derrumbándose.* Anagrama, 2022.

Sánchez Cruz, Jorge. "Intimacy, Relationality, Repair: AIDS, Mexico, and the Case of Agustín Martínez Castro." *Journal of Latin American Cultural Studies* 34, no. 1 (2025): 47–73. DOI: 10.1080/13569325.2025.2466436.

Sigma-Aldrich. 2019. "Product Information. Ripa Buffer." https://www.sigmaaldrich.com/deepweb/assets/sigmaaldrich/product/documents/350/775/r0278bul.pdf.

"U.S. Statistics." *Hiv.gov.* https://www.hiv.gov/hiv-basics/overview/data-and-trends/statistics.

Zaidenwerg, Ezequiel. "Néstor Perlongher y sus cadáveres: del neobarroso a la necropoética." *Cuadernos de Literatura* 19, no. 38 (2015): 432–49. DOI: 10.11144/Javeriana.cl19-38.npsc.

Perlongher's Bibliography

"A Viral Competition over AIDS." *The New York Times*, April 26, 1984, 22.

"Ainda Existe Vida Gay Depois da AIDS? As Assutadoras Mudanças nas Relações Homossexuais Masculinas." *Nova: Cosmopolitan*, March 1986.

Ariès, Philippe. 1974. *Western Attitudes toward Death from the Middle Ages to the Present.* John Hopkins University Press, 1974.

Assouline, Pierre ,and Pier Boncenne. "Les intellectuels, le SIDA et la realité." *Lire* 122 (1985): n.p.

Bell, Alan P., and Martin S. Weinberg. *Homosexualities: A Study of Diversity Among Men and Women.* Simon and Schuster, 1978.

Black, David. "The Plague Year." *Rolling Stone* 445 (1985): n.p.

Cardoso, David, dir. *Estou com AIDS.* Dacar Produções Cinematográficas, 1986.

Carrara Sergio, and Claudia Moraes. "AIDS: Um virus só não faz doença." *Comunicações do Iser* 4, no. 17 (1985): n.p.

Castells, Manuel. "Cultural Identity, Sexual Liberation and Urban Structure: Gay Community in San Francisco." In *The City and the Grassroots: A Cross-Cultural Theory of Urban Social Movements.* University of California Press, 1984.

Clavreul, Jean. *A ordem médica: Poder e impotencia do discurso médico.* Editora Brasiliense, 1983.

del Cabral, Manuel. *El escupido*. Editorial Quintaria, 1970.

Deleuze, Gilles, and Félix Guattari. *A Thousand Plateaus: Capitalism and Schizophrenia.* Translated by Brian Massumi. University of Minnesota Press, 1980.

de Sade. Marquis. *Philosophy in the Bedroom.* Translated by Richard Seaer and Austryn Wainhouse. Publishers Group West, 1975.

Dupin, N., M. Grandadam, V. Calvez, I. Gorin, J.T. Aubin, S. Havard, F. Lamy, M. Leibowitch, J.M. Huraux, J.P. Escande, and H. Agut. "Herpesvirus-like DNA Sequences in Patients with Mediterranean Kaposi's Sarcoma." *The Lancet* 345, no. 8952 (1995): 761–62. DOI: 10.1016/s0140-6736(95)90642-8.

Folha de S. Paulo: Um journal a serviço do Brasil 25, no. 20,549 (July 1985): n.p.

Foucault, Michel. *History of Sexuality.* Vol. 1: *An Introduction.* Translated by Robert Hurley. Pantheon Books, 1978.

———. *The Birth of the Clinic: An Archeology of Medical Perception.* Translated by A.M. Sheridan. Routledge, 1973.

Fry, Peter, and Edward Mac Rae. *O que é homosexualidad.* Editora Brasiliense, 1983.

Friedan, Betty. "The Happy Housewife Heroine." In *The Feminine Mystique.* Dell Publishing Co., 1970.

Gallo, Robert C., Syed Z. Salahuddin, Mikulas Popovic, Gene M. Shearer, Mark Kaplan, Barton F. Haynes, Thomas J. Palker, Robert Redfield, James Oleske, Bijan Safai, Gilbert White, Paul Foster, and Phillip D. Markham. "Frequent Detection and Isolation of Cytopathic Retro-viruses (HTLV-III) from Patients with AIDS and at Risk for AIDS." *Science* 224, no. 4648 (1984): 500–503. DOI: 10.1126/science.6200936.

Genet, Jean. *Querrelle.* Grove Press, 1974.

Gorin, Isabelle, Odile Picard, Liliane Laroche, Jean-Paul Escande, and Jean Hewitt. "Kaposi's Sarcoma without the U.S. or 'Popper' Connection." *The Lancet* 319, no. 8277 (1982): 908. DOI: 10.1016/S0140-6736(82)92176-6.

Illich, Ivan. *Medical Nemesis: The Expropriation of Health.* Pantheon Books, 1976.

"Medicina e Saúde." *Istoé* 9, no. 474 (1986): 38–39.

Miller, David, Don J. Jeffries, John Green, J.R. Willie Harris, and Anthony J. Pinching. "HTLV-III: Should Testing be Routine?" *British Medical Journal* 292, no. 6525 (1986): 941–43. DOI: 10.1136/bmj.292.6525.941.

Montagnier, Luc. "A History of HIV Discovery." *Science* 298, no. 5599 (2002): 1727–28. DOI: 10.1126/science.1079027.
Montero. Paula. *Da doença a desorden*. Graal, 1985.
Pollak, Michel. "A homosexualidade ou: A felicidade no gueto?" In *Sexualidades Ocidentais,* edited by Phillipe Ariés and André Bejin. Editora Brasiliense, 1985.
"Saudável negócio: A corrida da cura da AIDS tem cifras millonárias." *Revista Veja* 898 (1985): 132.
Sontag, Susan. *Illness as Metaphor*. Farrar, Straus and Giroux, 1978.
Samuel Sion, Fernando. "Dossier AIDS." *Ciencia Hoje* 5, no. 27 (1986): n.p.
Schemla, Elizabeth. "Sida: la tragédie africaine." *Le Nouvel Observateur* no. 1157 (January 9, 1987): 39–40.
SIDA booklet, edited by the team of the Pasteur Institute of Paris, coordinated by Dr. Montagnier. Foundation Interationale pour l'Information Scientifque, Paris, October 1985.
Silvério Trevisan, João. *Devassos no paraíso.* Editora Record, 1986.
Tronca, Italo A. "Historia e doença: a partitura oculta (A lepra em São Paulo, 1904–1940)." In *Recordar Foucault,* edited by Renato Janine Ribeiro. Editora Brasiliense, 1985.

www.ingramcontent.com/pod-product-compliance
Lightning Source LLC
LaVergne TN
LVHW022008200926
848481LV00007B/2290
9781685713454